To; John,
Best of luck
to a fellow

TONY NATURALE
"LET'S TALK FITNESS"

Senior Ball Player

Ty Natal

TONY NATURALE
"LET'S TALK FITNESS"

Anthony V. Naturale

Two Harbors Press
212 3rd Avenue North, Suite 570
Minneapolis, MN 55401
612.455.2293
www.TwoHarborsPress.com

ISBN - 978-1-935097-13-6
ISBN - 1-935097-13-x
LCCN - 2008909340

Book sales for North America and international:
Itasca Books, 3501 Highway 100 South, Suite 220
Minneapolis, MN 55416
Phone: 952.345.4488 (toll free 1.800.901.3480)
Fax: 952.920.0541; email to orders@itascabooks.com

Cover Design by Jenni Wheeler
Typeset by Peggy LeTrent

Printed in the United States of America

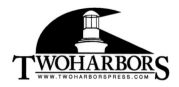

CONTENTS

IN MEMORY OF DOCTOR DONALD H. SLOCUM

If DOCTOR DON is listening now, I'm going to ask him to put his mighty catcher hands over his ears because, to me, he was the most everyday-kind-of-guy-genius I have ever met in my life; a man who stood both of and above his age and had the gift of breathing life into what is best in every living person. In all ages there have been some excellent workmen, and some excellent work done, but he was a mosaic of all of us.

To be wise, funny and an athlete is a rare combination, but he made playing baseball an everyday art for all of us, keeping us young in spite of our knee and hip replacements, waning vision and aching muscles; all the while charming us into believing we would hit another home run. None of us could deny him and we drew from all those youthful years on sandlots across America. He would not let us grow old and miss catching a falling star.

Three years ago when I began my journey of this book, Doctor Donald Slocum was in excellent health, a great athlete and a great man whom I am proud to have known. He wrote words of wisdom in my first book and he also wrote in this book. He accomplished so much in his eighty years, including inventing CORIAN, the hard counter surface top; ran the senior Olympics baseball and softball teams and actually played in them. He authored many books and periodicals and much, much more. I could write a book on Doctor Slocum and maybe someday I will.

This book is dedicated to you, Doctor Don, and I know you are probably creating a team somewhere in the clouds. Some sunny day I know we will meet again.

Thank you, Doctor Donald Slocum, not just from this author, but from all the baseball guys and all the people who were fortunate enough to have crossed your path. I remember when you said: "All we need is some sun-warmed grass and a little dirt under our spikes to spend one more day playing baseball. Baseball – it saved my life." And thank you, Barbara Slocum, for lending your husband to so many of us.

ANTHONY NATURALE

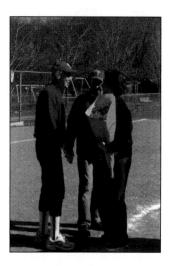

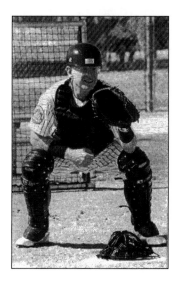

Al Overbaugh and Joe Crofton, players, presenting flowers to Barbara (Mrs Donald Slocum) before a cancer benefit game, in memory of her husband Doctor Donald Sclocum,. in Randolph N.J. April 2008.

Dr. Don catching the baseball at age 79.

AUTHOR'S COMMENTS

Welcome to Tony's World! Somehow I knew, sooner or later, I don't know why and I don't know how, but I knew you would find me. Actually I have been waiting for YOU! Yes, YOU!

I'm tired of telling my wife I don't need anything for Christmas or my birthday because my waist is the same as it was when I was in the United States Navy. Of course I am a gym-in-the-making and have been 24/7 for the past 50 years and then some. I told my wife I had to leave the marital bed because of her snoring when, in reality, I didn't want to disturb her rest doing the 400 sit-ups I do daily. We compromised, though, and I moved back in and do them on the floor as our cat Molly waits to watch me.

I know, I know, I am a pain in the neck as I am always giving advice to young and old alike, but they listen as they see me, over seventy-six, playing softball four times a week unless there is snow on the ground; not to mention I bowl twice a week...but this is about YOU!

Okay, you have opened this book and are obviously interested in getting fit, but if you think you are going to get your own program and exercises to make you an Adonis, you better close the book right now, because that's not what this tome is about.

It is the life story of many people–policemen, firemen, doctors, nutritionists, dancers, students, ball players and even me–doing things to give you a better life. Most of us have been through the mill and have tried everything, and at the age of some of us, that has covered just about everything. So you see, you are getting the opportunity to eliminate a lot of the time and steps many of us have wasted throughout the years, in an attempt to get fit and enjoy a better life.

And you youngsters can benefit too by learning some tricks from us "oldsters." We didn't become fit at this age by just sitting around and playing computer games and watching television.

The best way to get in shape and stay fit is to digest the following interviews from persons from all walks of life who have gone through it, and change your bad habits so you can have a positive healthy life.

The ages vary from the youngest at seventeen to the oldest at one-hundred – yes, that's right, one-hundred years old (my beautiful Aunt Margaret Farano), but most all of the interviewed are senior citizens.

We did the talk and we did the walk, so if you think you are qualified, then read on and see if you can do the walk and find your "Field of Dreams"… I FOUND MINE AND MANY OF THE PEOPLE INTERVIEWED HAVE FOUND THEIRS. GOOD LUCK AND I'LL SEE YOU ON "YOUR FIELD OF DREAMS."

Anthony (Natch) Naturale

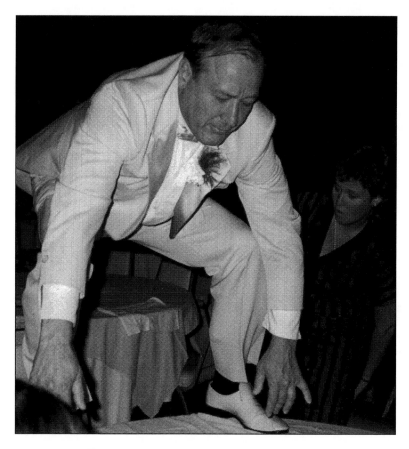

The author, at age 60, doing his famous table jump

DISCLAIMER: The contents in this book are my opinions only and the comments of the people interviewed cannot be verified, but I trust them as I hope you will trust me.

MADELINE'S COMMENTS

(My wife – I do trust her)

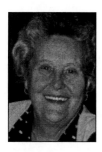

The author's wife, Madeline.

Let's have a moment of silence please as I welcome you, via the written word, into "Anthony's World of Fitness."

Before I begin, you need to know that "once upon a time" I was surrounded by handsome, athletic and intelligent men who just happened to be my brothers...five of them, plus my big daddy; they were all ready to protect their little spoiled sister at the drop of a dime.

Let's just say that after fifty-one years of marriage, I believe I am the only one who calls my husband Anthony... and for good reason: he is a focused, fanatic fitness guru who has never, ever let up on trying to keep me ready to try out for the Olympics, a woman's softball team or a dance marathon. This man was so different than my siblings I became fascinated, and still am, with the man, and yes, he is a fitness fanatic.

How do I know that? Just bear with me a little bit and I'll give you some history.

I saw him run in a three-mile race when he was over fifty-five years old. He was running so hard at the end so he could beat out a ten-year-old kid (the kid was in really good shape). He did beat the kid out.

He plays baseball and softball three times a week and bowls two times a week. I have watched him dance for hours at a time, never leaving the floor – never tiring – and usually dancing with women thirty years younger than he. (No, I'm not jealous – better them than me.) I watched him work two jobs just about all our married life. When he worked as a police officer on the 12 midnight to 8 a.m. shift, he would change clothes when he got off, and then go work with the electrician for four to six more hours. When he worked the 4 to 12 p.m. tour, he would start the side job at 8:30 a.m., come home sometimes as late as 3 p.m., shower, get into his uniform and make it into the police station by 4 p.m. When he worked the day shift, some of the days he would get home at 4 p.m., go work for a few more hours, sometimes getting home as late as 10 p.m., shower, go to bed and then start over again. Oh yes, and some of those days in between he would work out with the weights in the cellar to stay in shape and a heavy punching bag that used to shake the floor when he hit it. I used to yell at him till doomsday…he never heard me and just kept punching. And oh yes, he also attended and graduated from Montclair State College from age forty to forty-five somehow in between all of this activity. He always said to me he had to be in better shape than the criminals (and he was).

He is a man who is constantly in motion. He would place this chinning bar between the doorways (usually ruining the woodwork) and do pull-ups and chin-ups. At age seventy-six he still thinks nothing of doing push-ups during the commercials of a TV show and constantly doing isometrics all day long. He makes me tired just watching him. Would you think he is a fanatic? Well, you know what my answer is – watching this for over fifty years, it's an emphatic yes. It seems like nothing to me now. He constantly tries to get me to exercise, but so far he hasn't succeeded. He does, however, attempt to get me to eat right, and I have to admit it has helped me. Although I don't like oatmeal every day, I will have it from time to time. He makes me breakfast almost every morning and always puts a few apricots and prunes on the tray and, during the few days when he is home, is constantly pushing nutritious snacks on me. He has convinced me to eat better, and I love his Fig Newtons (thanks, Anthony).

Will I read his book? Of course I will, and I may even listen to him a little more (about getting into shape only).

Luv ya, Antnee... —*Madeline*

Anthony answers: Yes, I guess I am a fitness nut. I am neither a doctor nor a health expert. Many of the suggestions in this book are derived from different experts via books I have read, but most of it is the process of doing and eliminating over my lifetime. One very important aspect is what works for one may not work for another, but it has worked for me, and it is my sincere hope that it will work for you if you follow good eating habits and exercise regularly (and read my book). So follow me on this journey into good health and better living.

ACKNOWLEDGEMENTS

I would like to acknowledge all the once-healthy, soon-to-be-again people all over the world I see walking around every day, for they have given me the incentive to get in shape, stay in shape and to write this book. I'm not kidding... this is my quest, my journey that keeps me going in the hopes we can all benefit and enjoy life with our mates and watch our grandchildren grow up.

Then there is my wife, Madeline, my mate for over fifty years. She would get me so aggravated I would go down into the basement and exercise, so thank you, Madeline, and thanks to the really fast-running criminals who proved to me I had better run faster than they did or they would get away with their respective crimes.

Most of all, I would like to thank my mom – she instilled in me, at a very early age, to exercise and be active. She would listen religiously on the radio – we didn't have TV then – to a guy named Gaylord Hauser, a nutritionist, and a little later on to Jack LaLanne. She was a big advocate of them. She would listen and do exercises with them while making breakfast for us in the morning. Everyone thought she was a little crazy then, but she was actually way ahead of her time. She was a bundle of energy. Thanks, Mom...

And thank you, God – You have given me good genes and allowed me to live long enough and have the perseverance to continue to exercise and eat right, but most of all to believe in myself.

PRELUDE

Like everything else about my life, nothing is as obvious as it first appears. One thing I was always able to count on was watching, at a very young age, my mother do all these crazy exercises.

Throughout the years, staying fit was imbedded in me and now, at the age of seventy-six, I wish to impart my findings to others.

Today's advertisers continue to push all sorts of pills and gimmicks to the public to stay fit and lose weight, and every day you read something different about what's good for you and what isn't. It seems to change constantly. All too many people are falling for the garbage you read and watch on TV.

This book is not about gimmicks, but common-sense activities I do and other people that I interviewed do, that will assist you both mentally and physically on your road to good health. I will impress upon you to believe in yourself because you can, and will, accomplish almost anything you dare to dream. My motto: "I believe I can and I believe I will." And so can you, young or old. Age is not a factor.

FOREWORD

by Grange (Peggy Rutan) Habermann

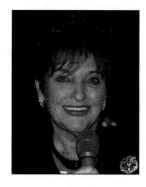

Grange Habermann

You guessed it: Tony Naturale has written another book – this one about fitness the "Naturale" way. And my book, *DEATH OF A BEBOP WIFE* by Grange "Lady Haig" Rutan, has finally been published (after fifteen years) about my first husband: Al Haig, the chosen pianist of Charlie Parker and Dizzy Gillespie, and later Stan Getz.

I told Tony, "Tony, I don't have time to introduce your book or to be your agent any more…it's my time…sorry."

Tony, giving me a deaf ear, closed his eyes, pretending not to hear me.

Focused and firm that Tony would listen, I appealed to his first friend from childhood, DONALD STAKE.

"Why don't you ask Donald Stake, your life-long buddy who wears Rockports and bermudas whenever you travel and you both look like the Bobbsey Twins? Let's face it, Tony, Donald's Swedish DNA qualifies him to be fit just by breathing and you are number one on his cell phone! He was your first 'Tribute' in *You'll Never Believe It* and your Best Man."

And, ever-the-cop-till-the-day-he-dies, as well as the athlete who never stops running up and down stairs during commercial breaks while watching the New York Mets and episodes of "Law and Order," he would not take "no" for an answer.

I tremble as I dare to tell you how he convinced me to step back into his healthy world: his desire to reach out and help people who have given up on trying to stay fit (as they are wooed in this world of fast food/packaged food with extra carbs and calories) is so strong he just keeps keeping on. Tony is the capo di tutti of facts and trivia on how to keep us all believing we can be young, fit and ready to live another hundred years.

The retired lieutenant put blinders on his ears and zap, wrote a review for my book, which came in the mail this morning. I felt his honesty, integrity, savvy, and know-how jump right out of the Internet, and here I am, once again, wanting you to take a ride via the written word as he gives you his inside skinny on becoming the best you can be...and with laughter. And you will see that "Tough Tony" sees life from the inside, the outside and across the board with the clarity necessary in this life to survive. And you know what? He knows how to eat, too – he has gained all of three pounds over fifty-five years – he was 195 and has ballooned to 198. Hmmmm, maybe he knows what he's doing.

Tony knows I don't have time and have been traveling back and forth to Las Vegas, Nevada for my book launch and arranging my own official signing at Barnes & Noble in the fall, but "super sleuth" will be a cop till the end and will not give up. So here I am, delivering, like he did for me when he was the first police officer at the scene of the D.O.A. at 999 Valley Road in Upper Montclair, New Jersey on that early morning on October 9, 1968. (This alleged murder is the crux of my book.)

Somehow, Tony Naturale seems to think that to change one's life you just start immediately, and there is no exception. Just bite the bullet and figure out a way, unique to you, and do it. Zap! I don't believe it. He says it is easy and there are no exceptions, anyone can do it. And this book is going to set the reader on a road to fitness.

Although there are answers to most of life's problems – for years I have tried to figure it out, but Tony always seemed to be on the cutting edge of staying fit while the rest of us were just wondering which way to go. He seemed to invent himself into a maverick of fitness without even leaving his home. In a day and age when there were advertisements in the back of magazines stating, "Don't let someone kick sand in your face, lift weights, drink the drink," he belts out with a smile, Tony seemed to know exactly what to eat, how much and why, when we had not even dealt with the question. The fact that he had twelve cars in his driveway and the Motor Vehicle Bureau said, "One more and you are a car lot" had nothing to do with the fact he was in top shape and fighting in the Diamond Gloves at the age of seventeen. Aside from being a great athlete, what did he know that I didn't know?

Perhaps I have the answer, as I witnessed his mother shaking wheat germ into ground meat when making meatballs or doing karate kicks at the sink and lifting her leg up onto the table for a good stretch as she bounded, bigger than life, through her busy day. Why, I was barely fourteen years of age when she gave me passes to a place in Montclair called, of all things, "Slenderella." I still remember this place, next to Bragg's Men's Store on Church Street in Montclair, where there were darkened booths and tables that rotated and jiggled me into laughter. Tony was brought into being fit through heredity, and I'm sure Josephine Naturale is looking down on her son and counting the reps.

Without further ado, I give you the man who keeps us all fit, because I was his agent and edited his first book, which is still doing quite well: *You'll Never Believe It* (the name of the book). But because we both grew up and graduated from Montclair High School and have known each other for over fifty years, here I am. Hey, what are friends for? Besides, I trust him because he once taught fitness at the Police Academy in Cedar Grove and would start every class with jumping up on the desk and introducing himself as the "Half-donut Lieutenant" – and they listened and lost weight and got in shape – even though he is not a fitness guru. I have seen the results of how he has helped many people from all walks of life and all ages. I have danced with him for hours at a time and he does not get tired (but then, I don't either, but I am much younger); he plays softball and baseball three times a week as long as there is no snow on the ground, participates in tournaments and is about to captain a team of over seventy-five-year-old athletes, sponsored locally, in Montclair, New Jersey, for the Senior Olympics being held in Kentucky in June of 2007.

[Note: They played and won all four games, winning the Gold Medal – nice going, NEW JERSEY EMBERS.]

Considering the reality his lovely wife, Madeline, is an excellent cook, he has defied the odds. When asked how he has stayed in such great shape, he innocently replies, "Motion and believe in yourself, that's all."

I said I don't have time, but I know I will read his book, and just maybe you will read mine.

Sorry, Tony, I cannot be your agent any longer, but – well, maybe – but not for a while.

Grange Rutan Habermann
Author of *Death of a Bebop Wife*
Cadence Jazz Books
www.amazon.com
www.ladyhaig.com
alhaigbebop@aol.com

CHAPTER ONE

ABOUT THE AUTHOR

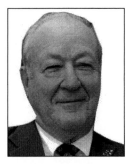

The author today (2008)

Many people have said to me, "Tony, you're not a doctor, a nutritionist or an expert on physical fitness, so why are you writing a book on it and why should anyone even listen to you?"

My answer: You're right, I'm just an average senior citizen, a guy doing whatever it takes to live longer and stay fit. I take no medication and still am in pretty good shape. I have stayed in this shape via the readings of other experts and through actual doing.

I am an "exercise nut" but most of all, I believe in what I am doing and I feel I can help other people in my age group – other average people – get in shape...motion is the key, so move it or you will not lose it (the weight).

As a police officer for over thirty-four years, I found out very early you had to be in better shape than the criminals you are chasing. It sure helped. It's one reason why when everyone was jogging, I did sprints. Many a thief was surprised when I apprehended them, that I wasn't a "doughnut-eating police officer" and could still run in my fifties. (Not all police officers are out of shape and eat doughnuts.) You see it seems to have worked for me and maybe it will work for you, too. Try it – you have nothing to lose except maybe a few pounds, and you don't have to run sprints.

So read on if you dare, and good luck – and if you're not a senior, you don't have to put this book down. Remember, you will be a senior someday. To me age only means "experience," so I guess I have seventy-five years plus of experience. (I keep changing that number. I was seventy-three when I started this book.)

My first book, You'll Never Believe It, is selling well. It took me almost three years and a lot of hard work, so why would I even take the time to venture into another book at this age?

I'm really not sure why, but I do know I want to do it and I have been somewhat fanatic about health and fitness all my life, so, why not?

Statistics in 2007 show that over 60% of American people are obese, and compared to other countries we are near the very bottom. That alone should give you incentive to get off of the obese list.

My mother exercised well into her seventies and she jitterbugged with me on her 78th birthday; having a mother who exercised instilled habits I carry on to this day…like mother, like son, I guess, as I am still doing 400 crunch sit-ups and 50 push-ups daily (no, my mother didn't do push-ups or sit-ups). I also learned some karate exercises many years ago which are incorporated into my daily routine. Mom didn't do karate either.

Okay, okay, so I'm very active and do my exercises daily. Big deal: A lot of people do and they aren't attempting to write a book…so why am I?

Well, I feel, and believe, I can aid and influence other people to get started on a simple exercise program. If anyone, at any age, puts their mind to it, they can help themselves by getting into a program…and it's healthy, too. So why don't you take this journey with me and decide if you want to begin to live longer and move your body, or just sit in the big chair and watch TV…or better yet, go to the fridge and grab some ice cream – that would be a lot easier than doing some exercises wouldn't it? And it would taste pretty good, too.

Everything I've learned has been through reading and

2

listening, but most of all through doing – in other words, my life experiences...and I've had many of them. You might say, "I'm a jack of all trades but master of none," which adds up to...I'm not a pro on exercise and nutrition, just an "average guy" doing whatever it takes to stay fit. In this book I have assimilated my knowledge, other people's knowledge that I interviewed, and my readings of other experts into my workouts. And you know what? It seems to have worked for me – at least that's what many people have told me. Of course you can't believe everything you hear, so you will have to keep on trying and experimenting until you find what works for you; kind of like "the process of elimination." In seventy-six years I've done a lot of eliminating. Hopefully, I've eliminated the right stuff.

I would like to share some of the things I have ended up with so you won't have to do as much eliminating as I have had to do. Just try it – you might like it, and if you don't – fuggedaboudit and go back to the couch and get some more ice cream from the fridge. Whatever you do, you can't help but improve yourself because you were off the couch for a little while, anyway.

In this book I have interviewed many people from all walks of life and they are telling their respective stories on how they eat, how they exercise and how they stay in shape. Some of the stories show how they have come back from serious illnesses and gotten back in shape. They have been "through the mill" and we can all learn from each and every one of them, so read on and learn how you can "get into shape" and live longer.

CHAPTER TWO

MY BACKGROUND

I would like to give you a little of my background so you know who you're talking to or who's talking to you. I am the son of Victor Naturale, who was born in Bella, Italy on January 22, 1905. He met my mom, Josephine Lemongelli (yes, that's how you spell it), who was born in Camden, New Jersey on June 8, 1912; they married in 1928 (yup – she was only sixteen…I think they named a song after her – kidding). I was born in Orange, New Jersey, on December 19, 1931. I also had a sister, Marie, and have a brother, Victor Junior.

When I was six years of age we moved from Newark to Upper Montclair, New Jersey, where I then attended Watchung, Mount Hebron and graduated from Montclair High School; I attended and graduated, when I was forty-five-years-old – I started at age forty – from Montclair State College. (It's now a University.) In fact, I'm qualified to teach history and social studies, which I just about passed in high school… Many of my high school classmates find this hard to believe, but it's true – honest. By the way, I am also Montclair High School 1950's class historian for our class reunions. The other reunion members voted me in to this (no one else wanted to do it). Some of my classmates still don't believe that.

I was in the United States Navy during the Korean War, from 1951 to 1955, and served on the Sibony, Valley Forge and the Midway…all aircraft carriers, and was honorably discharged as a third class petty officer. While a petty officer, I worked shore patrol and really loved it – I guess that's why I ended up a police officer for the Township of

5

Montclair, New Jersey. In the Navy I was very active, playing baseball, did some boxing for our ship, learned a little judo and lifted weights quite vigorously. I guess this kind of set the stage for my active life.

When I was discharged from the Navy, I worked for Bob Frei Electric for about one year. I then joined the Montclair, New Jersey Police Department in February 1956, and retired in 1990.

I was the first ever Internal Affairs Officer and Gambling Control Officer for the Township and after thirty-four years, retired as a Lieutenant and Watch Commander for the day shift. Following retirement, I became the Director of Safety and Security at a local hospital from 1990 to 1994. Today I am fully retired (I think).

I stated I was very active and I am; I play a lot of softball...I play two games on Tuesdays, practice on Thursdays and then two more games on Saturday; some of us seniors also play baseball on Wednesdays and sometimes practice baseball on Thursdays. Of course if we play a baseball game on a Thursday, there will be no softball practice on those days. We play from March until December or until the first snow.

Some women are golf widows; my wife is a baseball and softball widow. (I don't play golf – the ball is too small.)

I've played on the New Jersey softball Senior Olympics team, which plays all over the country. I've been to the last four Senior Olympics. The Senior Olympics is held every two years on the odd year and in a different state each year. We just came back from Pittsburgh this year (2005), winning the Bronze Medal in the seventy-and-over softball. Our seventy-five-year-olds won it all (Gold Medal).

In 2007 the Senior Olympic Games will be held in Louisville, Kentucky. God willing, I will be there and playing in the seventy-five-and-over competition. (NOTE: I'm still alive and did play in the Senior Olympics June 22-24, 2007 in Kentucky, and our New Jersey EMBERS 75's men's softball team won it all. Yup, we won the GOLD MEDAL, winning all four games. I was fortunate enough to be elected captain of the team (a picture of the team will be in the book). NICE GOING, NEW JERSEY EMBERS.)

In 2009 the Senior Olympics will be in San Francisco and 2011 in Houston, Texas, and God willing I'll be there, but let's not go too far into the future.

In the fall, and part of the baseball season, I bowl two nights a week, Mondays and Wednesdays, so during that period of time it's a very busy week.

I believe that many people don't have enough physical activities and that's why we, as Americans, are so obese. In fact, the last statistics have shown that the U.S.A. is the most obese country in the world, and they are claiming it's getting worse every day... We actually have it too easy. We have become very soft and because of the advancements of technology in our lives, television and video games, etc., we don't get enough exercise, and then there's all the junk food so many people eat.

So do you want to change this reality? Do you want to feel better? Do you want to extend your life so you can see your grandchildren grow up? Then get off your duffs and listen to this old guy. I'm not a professional anything and I didn't major in physical education or nutrition or anything similar to it, but I have been through the mill. I've tried everything from calisthenics to weight lifting, from boxing to karate, and anything else physical you can imagine. I didn't become a champion at any of them, but learned enough about all of them to evaluate what seemed best for me. I have also perused more health and nutrition books than I can count and have absorbed something from each and every one of them.

Every day I try something that helps me feel better physically. I have incorporated simple tasks into daily habits. For instance: running up and down the stairs instead of walking, doing dynamic tension and isometric exercises while I'm sitting down watching television. I know I look strange sometimes when I'm sitting down and pushing my hands together, one against the other, especially if there's a guest in the room, but those who know this strange "seventy-six-year-old fitness junkie" think nothing of it. The point I'm trying to make is you must incorporate the exercises you do into everyday habits and you can't go wrong. If you feel it's a chore, you won't continue it for too long.

I did teach Fitness and Health at the Essex County Police Academy in Cedar Grove, New Jersey for approximately two years, but that was the extent of it.

While there I became somewhat famous with my police recruits because I developed this "Table Jump." I would start the class sitting at the desk and before I even spoke, from the sitting position, I would place my hands on the top of the desk and simultaneously jump up onto the desk, ending up standing straight up on top of the desk... When I first started teaching a class to some older police officers I couldn't keep their attention, so I just jumped onto the desk and started giving my spiel. They seemed to pay more attention to me then, so I continued the rest of the class speaking from my desk top. I did this on impulse only and I held their attention, so when I started teaching to the new recruits, I did the same thing and it seemed to work. I was about forty-five-years-old at the time and most of the recruits were around twenty or so and seemed quite impressed that a man my age could jump like that (who was it that said white men can't jump?). Anyway, they seemed more inclined to listen to me. Most of the questions at the end of the classes were how a man of my age could jump like that and very little about the course itself; however, it was a lot of fun – and by the way, I still do the table jump, even with my knee replacement, but I am not recommending any of you to try this. I do it at special events like weddings, birthdays and reunions. (I did it at my Montclair High School 50th reunion and I hope to do it at my 55th.) My wife seems quite upset that I'm going to do it, but I told her all of my classmates, at age seventy-three, might not be able to see that well and I can just pretend that I do it and might get away with it.

Note: I didn't do it at my 55th – my wife said she would divorce me if I did and I hate to eat alone. I do plan on doing it at our 60th in 2010; by then I possibly may enjoy eating alone.

The fact is you can get into shape without resorting to this kind of exercise (jumping on a table). When people ask me how an old guy like me could jump like that, my pat answer was: There are three factors you need to be able to do this. (1) It's imperative that you have short legs. (2) You have to have a strong upper body. And (3) – and probably the most important – is you have to be a little crazy. Well, fortunately or unfortunately, I meet all the criteria.

The other thing I did with the recruits was have them (during coffee breaks) eat just half a doughnut, thereby consuming only half the calories during the break. Believe this or not, most of them did this. After a few classes I became known as the "Half a Doughnut Lieutenant." Well, you do whatever works, and I think it was worth it, because it worked. The most important thing was I was able to get through to some of the students who normally wouldn't have been listening to me. Actually I still come across some of the recruits that I trained and they remember me as "The Half-Donut Lieutenant." (See, they remembered something about my teachings.)

CHAPTER THREE

THE FIRST STEPS

I have often said I would not take advice from a bald barber on how to grow hair, but if that barber had a full head of hair, I might listen to some of his suggestions. All I'm asking you to do is listen to this seventy-three-year-old (probably seventy-six by the time I complete this book) experienced man. I'm not a Charles Atlas but I am in pretty decent shape and have been close to the same weight for over 50 years…so maybe I am doing something right. By the way, I don't have much hair – haven't found a good exercise to grow hair yet, but I'm working on it.

Now probably most of the people who are reading this book (who are not my relatives or friends) are seniors, but my concepts are actually for all ages, so don't feel bad if you're not a senior – you will be someday, so just keep on reading, no matter what age…and for you young oldsters, age is just a number. I call age experience. So are you ready? Then let's get started.

I'm going to start with some very simple steps for you to take that helped me, and a lot of the pros agree with them.

After you hear of my exploits, I will be interviewing mostly fit people to see what they do.

• TONY'S TEN STEPS •

1. Log everything you do as far as exercise goes and everything you eat – you will find as you go along it will help you tremendously, and you will probably be surprised at how much you actually shoved into

your mouth. You will see the daily improvement (hopefully) in black and white.

2. Exercise and Diet: Get into your head that you can't have one without the other. YOU MUST DIET AND EXERCISE – one will not benefit you much.

3. Possibly the most important thing to do is let your doctor know you are starting on a program, especially if you have some ailment that he is treating you for.

4. If possible, try and work your program with a friend. It's usually better if you're exercising with a buddy. You can encourage each other to keep it going.

5. Set goals at the beginning, i.e., I'm going to continue this for two months or three months or whatever, but you want to continue it, so don't set unrealistic goals.

6. The concept is to exercise before you eat – you will burn more calories that way.

7. Try and exercise the same time each day if possible or pretty much near that time. Of course if you can't, it doesn't mean you shouldn't exercise that day. Some days it may not be practical.

8. Try and eat five to six times a day – most experts believe this is better for your metabolism. I have personally done this for many years, even before I read it in the health books, and I'm a big advocate of this. They do not have to be regular meals. And do not have your main meal too late in the evening. I usually have a snack, like some fruit and nuts, as a meal. Some health experts recommend protein shakes, but I don't believe you need that much extra protein unless you are really into heavy weightlifting.

9. An important concept is to start a program – it doesn't really matter what program, but do something positive towards improving your overall condition. However, if you're already perfect, then stop reading

this right now and go back to the couch.

10. The last concept – and I believe it's the most important, that's why I left it for last – HAVE CONFIDENCE AND BELIEVE IN YOURSELF, AND SAY IT TO YOURSELF EVERY MORNING WHEN YOU WAKE UP AND START THE DAY: I BELIEVE, I BELIEVE, AND I BELIEVE. And you know what? You will start believing in yourself, and then you are on your way. Good luck.

• DOCTOR DONALD H. SLOCUM •

If you dropped Doctor Donald Slocum into the middle of the Sahara Desert, it would not take long for him to find seniors to make up a team to play ball. His thirst to have us all on that "Field of Dreams" is not quenched until he finds us. He does not need a phone or computer to find us, as there is an invisible grapevine that lets us all know he's looking for us…and we would follow him anywhere, because he has been one of the most inspirationally fit persons I have ever met. I have been playing ball with Doctor Don for over ten years now and every time I'm with him, I become more and more impressed. He is an author, inventor, lecturer, member of Who's Who, baseball and softball player, and organizer.

When I first met Don, he seemed to be running the entire softball and baseball leagues, and he actually was, with the help of John Healy, Walter Maly, Bernie Salinger, Sal DiBenedetto and a few others. I thought he was a medical doctor because he was always helping the ball players with their respective ailments. I asked him about my sore arm and he immediately prescribed solutions for it, and it worked, so why wouldn't I think he was a medical doctor?

Don also introduced me to baseball again in my late years, and get this: as a seventy-eight-year-old, he was the baseball catcher (one of the toughest positions in baseball) as well as the organizer, taking us to numerous baseball tournaments around the country. He also was one of the main organizers for the New Jersey Embers softball teams of seventy-five to seventy-nine-year-olds into the Senior Olympics. I never realized how much work this was until I was selected to do it this year (2007).

Don, while working for Hoffmann-LaRoche, invented the counter hard top surface "Corian," named after his young daughter, Corrie Ann. He is constantly traveling around the county lecturing on multiple subjects. At age eighty, Don has been the picture of health and I am honored to have Doctor Donald Slocum be a part of my fitness book.

Doctor Don wrote a speech addressing a college graduating class a few years ago, which illustrates how important it is to believe in yourself. Don had three positive concepts... Go, Don. Here's that speech...

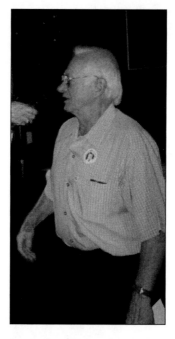

Doctor Donald Slocum at one of
his speaking engagements.

"First, remember your heritage. Not some ancestral aspect, but the totality of your life experiences: Your family,

14

friends, your teachers, preachers, and all your history, as they are a part of you. They belong to you and they are a source of your strength.

"Precept number two: Take care of your body. Keep it healthy and fit, because it is the vessel for your mind, your soul and your heart. It is these that make up your character, and that is certainly worth caring for. This will allow you to use your talents, putting them to work for the benefit of yourself and those around you. Creativity is nurtured by a healthy body and mind. Many times I needed to rely on endurance and stamina to give me strength on my journey to creative solutions.

"The third and final precept is: You must believe – first in yourself, then in life, and then in those values you cherish even now which as a youth sustained you to this pinnacle. And continue to believe. Even an inventor like Edison, or a theoretician like Fermi, or a Shakespeare, a Rembrandt, a Chopin, needed the confidence and surety of self to have accomplished what they did. I'm proud to say I've written many technical articles, been awarded numerous patents and introduced a number of commercial products; however, had I heeded the naysayers and listened to the skeptics, chances are I would have accomplished very little along the way. So remember – NEVER STOP BELIEVING."

Thanks, Doctor Don, not only for all that you have done for me and all the other ball players, but for your strong beliefs and how you have applied them to all of us. You are an inspiration to me and many others, not just ball players. See you on our "FIELD OF DREAMS."

CHAPTER FOUR

MY ROUTINE

NOW I'M GOING TO GO INTO HOW MY DAY IS, TO GIVE YOU AN IDEA, AND YOU WILL REALIZE WHAT A FITNESS NUT I AM... You don't have to be as nutty as me. Just get some ideas and remember...BELIEVE THAT YOU CAN AND YOU WILL.

I wake up whenever I feel like it (that's the advantage of being old and retired), unless of course there is something specific I have to do that day. My first exercise is to brush all my teeth, which I still proudly have – of course I do this very vigorously so I get some benefits from it (only kidding). I start by doing a lot of stretching, for about ten minutes, trying to stretch every muscle in my body, then get on the bedroom floor and do approximately 200 crunch sit-ups. One day I might do 50 from different angles so I get to the oblique muscles, usually doing 50 from each angle. Some days I may do sets of 30 each twice, so that would total 240 instead of 200. I try to vary it each day. I then do the karate kicks from the floor, both side and front kicks. I also do this in sets and sometimes do a straight 50. I always try and get at least 50, even if I do them in sets; however, in sets it will probably be 20 three times. I then lie on my back and stretch the back, bending my knees and bringing them to my chest, doing 50 or sets of 20 three times. I then lie on my stomach and work my legs, bending them towards my rear. This is very beneficial to me because I did have a knee replacement and need to keep the muscles in that area working. This all takes about twenty minutes and I'm basically done for the day until bedtime, when I will just do the 200 sit-ups before I retire...

Mondays, Wednesdays and Fridays I work out with 25-lb. dumbbells. I will do curls and triceps exercises and will do three sets of 15. If I really feel good I will do four or five sets, but the usual is three sets. If it feels too light, I will increase the reps. Besides the curls and triceps, I don't know what you call these, but I lie on the bed sideways with my head hanging over the side and, using the same weights, drop them from my chest over my head and just about touch the floor. (I think they call these pullovers.) I will do three sets but with the same 25-lb. weights and usually will get seven to ten reps from this. From the same position I do the fly exercise with my elbows slightly bent, so the benefit is in the chest and back area and not a strain on the elbows. One important technique is to do them slowly so that you really feel it. This takes around twenty minutes or so.

Sometimes I will use my exercise bands, which you can buy for approximately $10. These are great for stretching and warming up but can also be used for a regular workout. I double them up and sometimes triple them to have more resistance, trying to keep the reps under twenty. These are great because you can take them with you and hang them on a bed post or stand on them and do curls and triceps exercises. Sometimes I will do a full exercise routine with just the bands. I try to change up from time to time. That's it as far as exercise goes. Oh, I forgot, I also do my brain exercises every morning – I do the *Star-Ledger* crosswords and the Sudoku, and my wife thinks I'm a genius. Of course I'm not, but why not let her believe it?

You're probably thinking right now – boy, that's not much to stay in shape, and you're right – that's not much, but just a minute. Do you think you're done? Do you think that's the whole program? Well, here's the real secret: It's what you do the rest of the day that's really important. If you work out a total of about an hour a day, that leaves 23 hours left (minus sleep time).

It's the little things you do the rest of the day that are really important. You have to be active THE WHOLE DAY.

And how do you do that? It's all just common sense. IF YOU DON'T MOVE IT, YOU WON'T LOSE IT (pounds, that is). REMEMBER THAT. Keep that body moving. When you are walking, try and swing your arms and use as many muscles as you can during your walk.

Earlier I had stated you should write everything down. This is so important in following through with any program, and even the experts agree with me on this – or I should say I agree with them. Write down what you eat – everything, even down to the water you drink – and also write down the exercises you did, even if you walked down to the mailbox. This is the only way you can evaluate yourself, so maybe the next day you may want to eliminate a piece of pie or a candy bar that is staring at you from your notes. (Whenever I eat something very sweet, I will capitalize it so that it sticks out in my notes.)

NOW I'M GOING TO CONTINUE ON WITH MY DAY.

I go downstairs and usually make myself oatmeal. I always add walnuts and raisins and bananas to it, to make it more nutritious. Of course I usually make my wife something too... Yep, that's right, guys, I make my wife breakfast almost every morning. I am slowly convincing her to eat better, but it's a tough job. I try and equate every chore to an exercise (I told you I'm fanatic), and when I make her coffee in the microwave I have two minutes; I will usually do karate kicks for that two minutes (I hate to waste time). Sometimes I will do dips on the dining room chairs, but not for two minutes – that's really tough to get more than ten to twelve a set.

Now we have a condo with four sets of stairs. I will run up and down the stairs – never walk. (I've spilled the coffee a few times.) One day I counted how many times I went up and down, and I believe it was 45 times. Of course that's not every day. Some days I don't have to bring my wife breakfast in bed – ha. (She wants me to delete this and I said I would, but I lied. What husband listens to his wife? I'm no different.)

Now the day continues, and if I'm not playing baseball or softball I might have a small electrical job to do, and that keeps me busy again running up and down cellar stairs. If I don't do anything physical that day I may stay home, be on the computer (exercising my fingers), or watching TV. Now if you were watching TV with me, you may really think I'm a nut because I will never watch a commercial. As soon as it comes on, I will run up the stairs and just move around, maybe get a drink of water or cranberry juice (once in a while I have something sweet like ice cream). If I have something really bad, the next commercial I will go in the garage and jump on my stationary bike for at least five to ten minutes.

On my off days when I don't use the weights, I have a Chuck Norris gym in my garage that I will work out on for about twenty minutes on Tuesday, Thursday and Saturday or Sunday. This machine is great for stretching as you are pulling against your own weight. My children had given me this machine for my 65th birthday; for my 70th they gave me a set of weights. I'm wondering what I will get for my 75th (if I'm still here).

Note: *Okay, I'm still here, and they gave me a computer chair. I wanted a new punching bag, but I guess I'll have to wait for my 80th birthday.*

CHAPTER FIVE

YOUR HABITS

Well, I think you are getting the general idea how motion is so important to keep fit. If you have it on your mind and you have it on paper, you can't fail. Circulation is the key to good fitness, and circulation is the key to a good social life, too (only kidding...). There are so many simple and commonsense things you can do to stay fit. How many times did you drive around in the parking lot looking for a spot right next to the doorway? You should try and park as far away as possible and walk to the store. You will feel much better physically and you will be breathing the good air as you walk.

This too is very important in your exercise program – your breathing. Make sure you breathe deep and exhale it all out so your lungs get the workout, too. Every night before I go to bed, no matter how cold it is, I open up the window and take deep breaths. Not only is this good for your lungs, you will find you will sleep much better. This isn't just me saying this; many of the pros agree with this. I was looking out the window and breathing in one night at our condo and there were a lot of other fit people sticking their heads out the window and breathing hard. It caused quite a breeze that night. (Only kidding...)

As you read this book, you are going to find out this is a little different than most fitness books. You will also find out I'm a little different, too, especially in my approach to fitness. I firmly believe that you have to incorporate exercise into your everyday activities so that they become "habits." It's like anything else in life. If you do something over and over again, it will formulate your habits and the exercise will not

21

become a chore. The main thing is you should believe in what you're doing and enjoy doing it. So I guess you could say you are doing "mental exercise" too.

My approach in this book is also going to be different because I will be interviewing different persons about their respective days and their approach to fitness. Some of these people will be experts in the field, and many will be just the average person on the street or wherever I catch them. Some will be tremendously out of shape, too. So watch out...I may even catch you, the reader, and look for your daily routine. You may not even be physically fit, but remember what I said earlier: we have to eliminate some steps we take to get to the proper fitness level, and some of the data you give me may be some of the elimination steps. So you see, no matter what you do for yourself or what you don't do for yourself, it will be a help. But don't ask me for a percentage in the book, because I'm not planning on making much money. I just hope that it will help some of you out there to improve your body.

Remember the song, "Everybody loves somebody sometime"? Well, I hope you love your body enough to keep it going a very long time so that you can see your grandchildren grow up.

CHAPTER SIX

THE INTERVIEWS

They told me a tree grew in Brooklyn, but did you know GEORGE BECK also grew up in Brooklyn? The guy from Brooklyn is first. Let's hear your story, George.

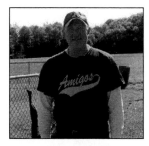

George Beck

Growing up in Brighton Beach, Brooklyn, was an easy place to become athletically active. The daily routine included coming home after school, immediately putting on "play clothes" and running back to the schoolyard at PS 225 to get into a game of softball, basketball, touch football, punchball, or stickball (with a broomstick and a burned tennis ball).

What game we played depended on the season and how many ballplayers showed up. We had the cement schoolyard and no easy access to baseball fields; hence, we played softball by choice. Sometimes we played hardball on cement, but this was only for the fanatics. When it got too dark to play (no lights in the schoolyard), we would move to the streets to play stoopball, punchball, or stickball under the street lights. We would grudgingly move out of the way for cars or if we were in the middle of a play, we would make them wait until they started blowing their horns, and then we might switch to Ringalario or Johnny on the pony. So you see, we spent much more time playing ball than anything else, except maybe sleep. In the fall we would play tackle football on the beach without equipment but nice soft sand to fall on. There was no Little League then, but there was the Daily Mirror League, where we played our games on a "real" field at Lincoln H.S. This was such an important part of my life that kept me in shape, out of trouble and provided many close and lasting friendships, some to this day.

The reason I went through the above was to indicate that playing ball was one of the most important things in my life, and I believe it set the pattern for me to stay active as much as possible, and I continue that to this day. In high school and college and the Army, I got a chance to play football and run track. Those were special times and I cherish them still. The combination of all these factors made me a "ballaholic," always on the lookout for another place to play.

When I felt it was time to move into the workout gym, I became sad because there was something missing in my life – a game, a time and place to leave the world behind and go for that win. Ball games also represented a natural state of affairs: the better team won, you gave it all you had, you would sweat and strain in the effort and get tired. It was always worth it. When I found out about the Senior Softball League, I was ecstatic and have played in this league for 10 years with a bunch of great guys whose love of the "game" has kept me young in thought, even though these bones don't move as well as they used to. I get rejuvenated every spring at the first softball practice, the return to the fields and running and throwing, catching and hitting, and my allegiance to the "rites of spring."

I turned 68 last month and I realize I've had to change my eating habits. I find weight control more difficult than ever before. One thing I am doing is being careful about the size of the portions I eat and will usually eat more often (between four and six times a day). This way I can eat an apple to curb hunger and stretch it out to the next time I eat. I've cut down on red meat and increased the amount of fish, fruit and vegetables. I try to drink at least five glasses of water a day plus a lot of other fluids. I've always eaten low-fat foods in all applicable categories and restrict the amount of sugar I ingest. I also try to use ginger and pepper as spices and green tea as a beverage; very little bread and it has to be whole grain. I fight the late-night munchies by eating dried fruit and a glass of red wine.

All of the above works only as long as I do my exercises two to three times a week, working up a heavy sweat.

Currently, I weigh 210 and at 5'11" I would like to get back to 195 pounds. That will be a good winter challenge for me at age 68.

Thanks, George. Hey, did a tree really grow in Brooklyn?

JERRY BOLAND

The next story isn't just a fitness interview; it's a human interest story about a person that I met while in the US Navy over fifty years ago. Many of us veterans often wonder about the people we lived with while we were so very young. Some veterans have very sad stories of buddies they lost during battle. I was very fortunate that during the Korean War I was on ships that never got to Korea. I served on the Siboney, Valley Forge and the Midway, all aircraft carriers. It was a good thing because I never actually learned how to swim (still don't know how). We were on the East Coast traveling to the Mediterranean and that area, and had been on alert many times but never made the trip where the battles were.

I have often thought about some of the buddies who I lived with for four years of my life and what's happened to them. Not too long ago I made contact with a former shipmate, JERRY BOLAND, via the computer. We talked over the phone and via the computer many times. I did get to see him, but unfortunately it was at his funeral.

My wife and I made the trip to Scranton, Pennsylvania, and met his family at the wake. I was so glad I had made contact before he passed away, because his son told me that my sending him my first book, *You'll Never Believe It*, which had many incidents of us during the Navy years, made him very happy, and before he died he constantly talked about our escapades in the US Navy.

At his funeral, I met members of his family and they were very appreciative to me for giving him some enjoyment in his final days. We all miss Jerry.

MOLLY CAGGIANO

Today I came across a young female 17-year-old who plays softball and lacrosse for Montclair High School. She is the granddaughter of a very good friend of ours and after talking to her for a few minutes, I realized I should get her story. I know earlier I said the interviews were from people between the ages of 33 to 100, but I think we should hear from a young athlete, and we all know we can learn from each other. So let's hear from MOLLY CAGGIANO. Go, Molly

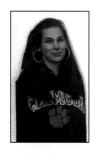

Molly Caggiano

I am a 5'8", 17-year-old junior at Montclair High School. Growing up as the only girl, I have always tried to keep up with my two older brothers (Michael and Bobby). They were very active in sports, playing football, baseball, and basketball. Since they played sports, so did I; I always wanted to keep up with the boys. I never wanted to be the one on the sidelines.

Today I play field hockey and softball for the high school. To keep in shape for these sports, I try to work out daily. I work out on the elliptical and the ab lounge and do different exercises to keep my arms, stomach, and legs toned. Whenever I get the chance, I try to go to Diane Tobin's spin class at the YMCA. It's an hour straight of cardio that has great music.

When it comes to eating, I am not one who diets. I try to eat right, but have a weakness for certain foods like my mom's steak sandwich, Keiko Naturale's pasta salad, and Carvel's ice cream cake with extra crunchies. I am not an expert on being healthy, but I say eat what you want, but keep the amount of what you eat reasonable. When it comes to being in shape, my goal is to be toned and have a lean body, and not to be "Miss Bulky."

Thanks, Molly, it's great to get the story from a young high school student. When you get to my age, I know you will still be in great shape.

STEVEN CANDIO

My cousin STEVEN CANDIDO, a former Cedar Grove policeman, has a pretty good story concerning his fitness. Go, Steve.

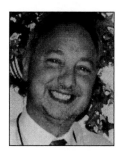

Steven candido

Growing up and while on the police department in Cedar Grove, I kept in decent shape – lifting, running and playing softball. Towards the end of my ten-year police career, I had ballooned to almost 200 pounds – height is around 5'7" – what with working nights and eating doughnuts (policemen love doughnuts). I've been practicing law the past eighteen years or so. Around eight years ago I evicted a gym owner on behalf of one of my clients. About six months later I received a call from another client who had moved and was storing 11 exercise work stations on behalf of a repossession company, coincidently from the same gym that I evicted. I sent a nasty letter to the repo company to pay their moving and storage charges. They called me and I convinced my brother Ken to purchase the equipment. He had no place to put it and I thought it would look good in my basement (and maybe I could charge him rent). It sat in my garage (too large to fit into the basement) for about six months when my neighbor and I decided to start using it. Over the years we have added additional weights and machines.

Around the same time I began running (more like walking). I would take my dog Jake (140-lb. yellow lab – big boned...honest) to the Cedar Grove HS track and run the straight-aways and walk the curves. When I hit a half mile

I felt I had accomplished something. There were mornings when my back was out of whack and I almost crawled to the track. Around the second or third lap I believe that the parts of my body were "oiled" and actually had my back/neck go back into alignment. I am now up to running about three times per week – usually 2 to 2.5 miles on weekdays and 4 to 5 miles on a Saturday or Sunday along the old Erie-Lackawanna railroad bed.

Feeling that I had finally gotten in decent shape, I have even run the Glen Ridge Ashenfelter 8K race, and would see these fat, old ladies passing me and about to finish a good 15 minutes before me! I am proud to say that I have gotten my weight down to around 170, and bench up to 300. I feel much better physically and will continue to exercise. I plan on seeing my grandchildren grow up.

Great job, Steve, and I know you will see your grandchildren grow up.

COL. BARRON J. CASTELLANO

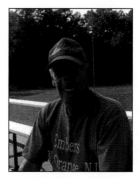

Barron J. Castellano

This next person, a fellow softball player, has had an illustrious career as a citizen-soldier. In a recent issue of the *Italian Tribune*, Col. BARRON J. CASTELLANO was recognized for his leadership excellence in both military and civilian public service. He was recently inducted into the Officer Candidate School (OCS) Hall of Fame at Fort Benning, Georgia. The honor was also awarded to such notables as Senator Bob Dole and Secretary of Defense Casper Weinberger.

Col. Castellano joined the NJ Army National Guard in 1949 at the Roseville Armory in Newark, NJ. He retired in 1985. In civilian life he served 25 years in law enforcement: seven years in the highway patrol, six years as undersheriff of Essex County, and twelve years in the Essex County Prosecutor's Office.

Barron is 78 years old and is still playing tennis and softball. He exercises six days a week, alternating three days of calisthenics/isometric exercises and three days of a light weight program, which are all performed in the early morning hours at a 45 to 50 minute duration.

Barron stated jogging and running are the best aerobic exercises, which he did for over forty years. Unfortunately, there was very little knowledge of training equipment and proper shoes at that time, which shortened his running career.

He tries to control his portions of red meat and eats very little food after dinner. He does take vitamins and supplements. He has two health mottos: (1) a piece of fresh fruit after every meal, and (2) everything in moderation.

Hey, Barron, it's been great playing ball with you all of these years, but don't forget the five movies you were in. What were they?

Barron answers: *The Godfather, The Sorcerer* with Roy Scheider, *Death Trap* with Michael Caine, *Cops and Robbers* with Joe Bologna, and an Essex County film on drugs, *The Retaliators.*

Wow, I'm playing ball with a celebrity, and it's an honor to have such an accomplished person as a part of my book. Thanks, Barron, and I'll see you on the ball field and maybe in the movies.

AL CHELI

AL CHELI has been playing ball with me a couple of years now and I like his "one-arm lift exercise." Let's hear it, Al.

At 61 I'm just entering "old age." More importantly, I'm one of the first of the Baby Boomers to reach that plateau. The Boomer Generation refuses to grow old.

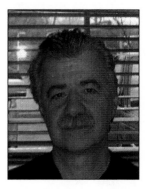

Al Cheli

We don't want to be called Senior Citizens, Retirees, Old Folks or anything like that. We are also the generation that made the act of exercising into an industry. It was during our watch that we all joined expensive gyms that we rarely visited and purchased expensive exercise equipment for our home that we rarely use. Collecting dust in my basement are a stationary bike, treadmill, rowing machine and a Bow something-or-other that looks like it could have been used in the Spanish Inquisition.

For most of my middle age I used an exercise routine that I learned earlier in life and perfected in college. One of those exercises is called the "Stationary One-Arm Lift." Place your elbow on a hard surface like a table with your forearm and hand facing forward. Place a small weight in your hand (a mug filled with a liquid works best). Lift the mug to your lips. Repeat until you become a little dizzy (or slightly drunk). It is important to remember to keep replenishing the liquid in the mug. It is not recommended that you do this exercise with both hands at the same time. This exercise is best performed while sitting down. (Also do not drive after this exercise.) I hope you all know I'm kidding; just a little levity.

In all seriousness, I wasn't a big exercise guy during my forties and into my fifties, and paid for it by gaining over 20 pounds. I now have a regimen of exercises that revolves around the "Ten Thousand Steps to Better Fitness" program. The idea of the program is to take at least 10,000 steps per day. I wear a pedometer throughout the day to count my steps. Most days I don't come close to the 10,000 steps. So what I also do is walk on the treadmill. Usually I wait until the evening to make up as many steps as needed. Here are some other ways to increase your daily steps:

Walk in place or pace when on the phone.

Get up during each commercial and walk around until the television program begins again.

Even better, walk in place during the television program.

Use a restroom that's farther from your office or on a different floor.

Take the stairs.

Walk around the mall while your wife shops.

Park farther away than you normally do.

Go to people's offices instead of using the phone or e-mail.

Take a walk at lunch and then eat at your desk.

In addition to the "Ten Thousand Steps to Better Fitness" program, I also do sit-ups each morning and a lot of stretching each day. I visit a "muscle release" specialist every couple of weeks to stretch me out.

Despite all this, I still haven't lost much weight. I still eat too much and too well. I've tried many different diets, none of which have worked very well. So my newest attempt to lose weight is hypnotism. The hypnotist leaves certain messages in your subconscious that are supposed to stop you from wanting to eat a lot and eat certain foods. I just started so it's too soon to tell if it's working. I also wanted my wife to see the hypnotist and make her think that I'm still young and sexy. He said he couldn't do that because he would need more to start with – I'm getting rid of him.

Good job, Al, but I think you have to look at some of the other interviewees in this book to increase your workout program. But

I like your sense of humor and believe me, that's also important for overall fitness. I think many of the other people in this book have used that one-arm lift. See you on the ball field.

STEPHEN DAGNO

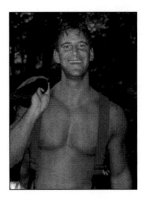
Stephen Dagno

Summer weather allows me to be exposed to a dip in the pool at our condo after a softball game in Wharton, New Jersey. Familiar faces become friends and an automatic "Hello" is the way my neighbors and I connect. Most days there is a very tanned "in shape" younger fellow who I think probably lifts weights. On a quest to include as many "fit" acquaintances and friends as possible in my book, I decide to interview this stranger, even though he is younger than most of the people I have interviewed and it is obvious fitness is a part of his daily routine. We begin to converse and I find out he's a Newark fireman and, "yes," he does lift weights, and works out regularly as well as swims. I ask him for an interview and he agrees to it. The following is from STEPHEN DAGNO, a Newark fireman.

Now you know you have to be in good shape to fight fires, especially in a big city like Newark, New Jersey, and that harsh reality keeps him ready to respond and protect 24/7 to handle the tremendous workload of carrying equipment and climbing up and down ladders. If you saw this 6'3" tall, 225-lb. fireman, you would immediately know he works out. Okay, Stephen, let's hear about your routine.

"My main workout is four workouts in a five-day period. I will work out with weights Monday through Friday with Wednesdays off. I try to keep each workout for approximately

45 minutes. I feel any longer than that could be dangerous to my joints. Each day I will work a different set of muscles, usually doing three sets of 11 to 15 reps with 30 seconds to one minute in between reps. After each workout I will do 120 sit-ups to cool down. If my workout does not exceed 45 minutes, I will fill in with other exercises to meet that time."

He is very careful with his diet, doing most of the cooking at the firehouse.

Steve did give me an extensive list of all the individual exercises he does and believe me, he does work all the muscle groups using weights.

Thanks, Steve, I know you will be around for a long time. It's good to know that someone who is protecting the citizens is in such great shape. See you at the pool.

ROLLIE DAX

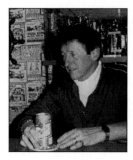

Rollie Dax

I have also been trying to get in touch with other shipmates (see Jerry Boland story), and just recently I made contact with ROLAND (ROLLIE) DAX. I met Rollie late during my tour on the Siboney (my last year on the ship) and we immediately connected. Rollie and I worked out together, went on liberty many times and seemed to have many of the same interests. Unfortunately, after only a few months I got transferred to the Valley Forge and I lost contact with Rollie.

The amazing computer has allowed me to again connect with Rollie, and the last few months we have been talking and passing photos back and forth. Rollie has had an amazing life, and when he told me he had 12 children, I immediately thought of the Montclair family (the Gilbreths) that had a movie made about their life, "Cheaper by the Dozen," and was quite a story. Well, I figured we should hear about Roland Dax's own "Cheaper by the Dozen" story from Wisconsin, USA, so let's hear it, buddy. Go, Rollie.

Well, Tony, like you I am also a fitness nut. It started when I was young. While in high school I played baseball, football and basketball, and I even boxed. It continued while in the Navy as I played on the ship's baseball team and was a catcher. When I played in Cuba, we would play for a barrel of beer.

My job kept me very busy – I was a "hook runner" on the flight deck and would greet the ships as they landed, and would be running on the flight deck while the planes were landing. They called this "hook running" as you had to un-hook the planes as they landed.

I also would pick up the captain from the airport to the ship and back to the airport. One amazing man, Captain Sears (I think he later became an admiral), was really very nice to me and I will never forget him. He treated me like an equal, and that is rare for commissioned officers to enlisted personnel. He actually let me take his commissioned car to go on liberty and left his hat on the front seat in case I got stopped. Fortunately I didn't.

Well, I know you're interested in my family because you know my wife and I have twelve children. Well, how about this? My mom and dad also had twelve children and my wife comes from nine siblings in her family. So you see, when we get together it's quite a mob. We have thirty grandchildren and fourteen great-grandchildren.

Because this is a fitness book, I have to say you must be active, as I was living in Wisconsin and working on my grandfather's farm as a young boy (we didn't have tractors then) and being very active in high school, playing sports and working out.

We started very early and the day after my wife turned sixteen, we got married. Nine months and a day after, we had our first child. By the time our first was two, we had four children. A few days later she turned three. In October 2008 we will be married for 54 happy years.

Raising a family of twelve has certainly kept my wife and me very busy.

Thanks, Rollie, you and your wife certainly have had an active and happy life. Good luck to you all and we hope to see you in the summer of 2008.

REMO DELLASANDRO

REMO DELLASANDRO is my neighbor and a police officer in Parsippany, NJ. He lives right across the street from me and I constantly see him punching the bag, lifting weights in his garage and jogging around the condo, so he must be in pretty good shape. Hey, Remo, what's your story?

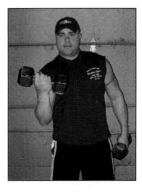

Remo Dellasandro

Well, being Italian, it's no secret that I love food, all foods from all cultures. It has been my downfall. I've been known to devour an entire pizza at one sitting. It's not a far stretch – growing up in a household where Sunday dinners could feed an army. My mother would often cook four pounds of pasta with mountains of meatballs for four people and insist that we have seconds (all Italian mothers do that). However, I love physical fitness as much as I love food, so in the early nineties when I fell in love with weightlifting, I had to combat these habits in order to see true gains.

I use pure motivation when I work out. When I see mentors like my father and Mr. Naturale, who are in their seventies and are in absolute excellent condition and constantly remain active, I find myself having no excuse for fatigue or laziness at the age of 32. At eighteen I enlisted in the Marine Corps, which in itself forces you to be physically fit. I left boot camp at 183 lbs. and maintained that throughout the years I spent in the Marine Corps. After I was discharged, I really hit the weights hard and without being forced to do cardiovascular activity, my metabolism drastically changed. I now weigh in at 240 lbs. (I like to think the majority of that is muscle) at a "towering" 5'9". I'm by no means a fitness expert and I have a long way to go for that "Adonis look," but through reading and other instructional tools, I know that the old saying, "you are what you eat," could not be more factual. Heavy weightlifting comes with a necessity to consume certain foods. A high-protein diet is the key to adding on lean muscle mass. Unfortunately, my aforementioned Italian heritage throws a huge wrench in that system. Whole pizzas are as beneficial to weightlifters as water is in your car's oil tank. I've tried every "quick fix diet" and various supplements. I have come to one conclusion... MOTIVATION. That's the number one factor, in my opinion, to achieving your fitness goals.

As a police officer, working a steady night shift, my choices for nutritious meals at work are few and far between, due to the fact there are three options: fast food, the greasy spoons and, of course, donuts (policemen love donuts). As a remedy, I prepare my own meals. Eating five to six well-balanced meals throughout the day is a key advantage to maintaining a high energy level to complete my workouts. Due to my work schedule, everything is in reverse. I sleep in the daytime and work at night. This, however, is only for four days at a time. Working four days and having four days off, when I have a normal schedule, takes an extraordinary toll on the body, both mentally and physically. There is one certainty: Nutrition is the only cure to function properly. I can see a drastic difference on the days I eat poorly as opposed to the days I don't. Therefore it is a must to take the time to prepare my meals far in advance. You can bench press 400 pounds but without the proper fuel, you are useless the remainder of the day. As any police officer will tell you, the statistics are not in our favor (especially if you work nights) for heart failure, high blood pressure, stress and obesity.

I almost never take any kinds of medication; therefore,

I have turned to a more holistic approach to health. I see a chiropractor regularly and try to ward off any ailments naturally. I recently began following a "blood type diet." Dr. D'Adamo recommends eating specific foods based on one's blood type. I'm an O negative, which means my body responds better to lean protein, such as dark meats like beef liver, kidney (I've yet to attempt that), dark fruits, and vegetables high in fiber. Virtually no simple carbohydrates are recommended in this diet. When I stick to this nutritional plan, it is evident how I get maximum performance out of my workouts. As Mr. Naturale may be able to attest to, being my neighbor, when I follow the "blood type plan," I can usually be seen doing vigorous training, such as running around my townhouse development wearing a 30-pound weighted vest or running repeatedly up the steep incline hill entering our development. In addition, I do a strenuous boxing workout or use the spinning bike at my gym for 45 minutes to an hour. Mostly, though, I stick to heavy weight training. I usually train one body part per day, with one or two days rest within the week. Legs and arms are my favorites, so I often spend more time on them. I don't make it a habit to record a maximum weight record, but last that I remember, I leg pressed 830 pounds and bench pressed 405. The bench press was about a year ago so I'm not sure if that's still an accurate record.

To sum it up, my training philosophy is this: four to six exercises per specific body part, consisting of five pyramid sets (including a warm-up set) of between 4 and 12 repetitions each, adding more weight each set, subsequently decreasing the repetitions. In addition, I'll throw in some cardiovascular and abdominal work. By the way, a strict nutrition schedule is paramount to getting that six-pack look. I've yet to get that look other than in my refrigerator, but maybe in Mr. Naturale's next book I will have conquered the pizza cravings and achieve that washboard stomach – who knows? As a side note, I always make sure I never use an elevator or park close to my destination.

I hope I'm on the right track with my routines and someday I might be as fit and active as Tony Naturale.

Thanks, Remo, that's quite a routine you have, and I have seen you running around the complex. When you get to my age, I'm sure you will have surpassed my fitness level, and I've done that eating a whole pizza thing too. My washboard look left me many years ago. Good luck.

SAL DIBENNEDETTO

Just a note about the next person I interviewed: SAL DiBENNEDETTO. He's an intelligent guy and an accomplished businessman and I also play ball with him, but remember I said not everyone I interview will be in shape or want to get in shape. But he has quite a story to tell. Go, Sam.

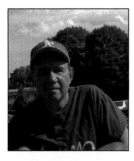

Sal Dibennedetto

<u>Preamble:</u> Trees, fresh air and sunlight. Life is a gift!

Why would anyone want to interview me on physical fitness? If the shoe fits, wear it... well, for me the "shoe" never did fit well.

I'm one of those guys who joins the YMCA, pays the $360 annual fee, goes for two or three weeks, and then completely stops going.

I'm one of those guys who begins the year with a resolution written on the refrigerator door...walk two miles a day.

For the first week or so, I walk two miles a day. Then I realize how cold it is and the warmth of my home affords me the opportunity to keep the front door locked and my winter coat in the closet.

I'm one of those guys who has his neighborhood teenager cut his lawn for twenty bucks. Then watch him through the living room window...sweating and swatting flying insects while going up and down across my front lawn.

I'm one of those guys who begins doing his stomach crunches in bed in front of the old TV, stopping at number

10 due to my interest in the CNN news.

Do I sound familiar to you?

I'm one of those guys who buys all kinds of vitamins and minerals at the local marketplace, and then neatly store the unopened bottle in a lower kitchen cabinet. I figure after one year that it's time to throw them out and go buy another bottle or two.

It's a family thing. My sister also hates exercising. I never saw my dad or my mother exercise, nor did I ever see my grandparents exercise. They must have had the same genetic make-up as I do. Therefore, at my age...70 years old, why even bother to think about it? I have no wrinkles, my hair is mostly black, and I have 20/20 vision. My pulse is between 50 and 60 beats per minute, I have low cholesterol and a very good memory.

Now, here's the kicker you've all been waiting for, right? For over 35 years, my career was as a food chemist. Hey, I can tell you a lot about food. Everyone knows that there's good food, not-so-good food and bad food, so why even discuss this subject?

Well, I've spent my entire life eating food. I think everyone who is reading this has, also. So, what's different about me, you say?

The job I had was a Quality Control and R&D research manager/director who specialized in tea. Yes...T-E-A.

I worked for a company that bought tea, processed tea and sold tea. They made billions and I got the "President's Award for Excellence." I wear that medal on my keychain. So much said for Corporate America.

Every morning one of the routines was "tea tasting." Prior to buying leaf tea from all over the world, it was one of my responsibilities to sample and taste hundreds of cups of tea each morning...before the real work day began, ugh! Little did I know that my body was absorbing all these antioxidants, 35 years worth!

Now, everywhere you go today you see the shelves stacked full with black tea, pekoe tea, and the newest of them all...GREEN TEA! Little Japanese men climbing the mountainside between tea bushes on television ads being asked "What is EGCG?"

After thousands of years of humanity drinking tea, we learn now that "green tea" is the newest health enhancer. Go figure.

The scientific claims are universal. It prevents cancer, lowers blood cholesterol, controls high blood pressure, lowers blood sugar, suppresses aging, aids in weight loss, and even fights tooth decay. Need a diuretic, drink tea.

It is truly a gift from Mother Earth. I drink almost a half a gallon of green tea a day. Here's how I brew it: I take a dozen tea bags and using two cups of boiling water, steep them for about ten minutes. I then remove the bags (after squeezing every drop of the golden brew), pour the liquid in a half-gallon container, fill it to the top with water, shake it and place it in the refrigerator to cool down. Sometimes, I squeeze a few lemons to get added flavor.

Whenever thirsty, I pour myself a glass full of green tea. Rarely is there any leftover green tea in a day. You can easily double this recipe.

NOTE: *I have added this last bit just recently because since I wrote the above, I have had a heart attack and am now recuperating.*

I was told that I should walk at least 30 minutes a day as part of my recovery program. Since I really don't like walking around the block for 30 minutes, I use my local supermarket and walk the aisles for over 30 minutes.

Today, while doing my exercise program at our ShopRite Supermarket, I noticed this young woman in her twenties and what she had in her shopping cart.

Obviously not into any diet or health program, I looked into her cart and saw the following:

Frito Lays, pretzels, Edy's ice cream, di Giorgio pizzas (2), cheese dips, salsa dips, cookies and a large cheesecake, two packs of sausage, whole milk, iced tea and an assortment of other high-calorie treats. Estimated over

20,000 calories in one carriage. She was about 5'7" and weighed around 110 lbs. A "Mia Farrow" look-alike.

Then I decided to check out this old man…around 75 years old. While he was browsing the shelves, I looked into his cart.

A large bag of grapes, fresh strawberries, navel oranges, mustard greens and collard greens, carrots, celery, miscellaneous vitamins and yes, CQ10 (a large bottle). I said to him that he really eats healthy and I admire his choice of wholesome foods. He stuttered, "Yeah, I eat healthy but I've had cancer, heart disease and arthritis eating this shit!" He was extremely thin and had difficulty walking with his cane.

So where is the middle ground? Ooops, there was this rather obese woman with her cart filled to the brim with all kinds of goodies. While she was selecting a pumpkin pie, I looked into her cart, also.

Well, 20,000 calories would be shadowed by over 100,000 calories of food stuffs. Man, this woman had every kind of food that would predict early burial. Atkins would turn in his grave if he saw what she was purchasing. However, she did have two bottles of Diet Coke buried under her White Castle cheeseburgers and kielbasi.

So, you're probably asking what I bought, right? Non-fat soy milk, yogurt, egg whites, lean veal cutlets, lean chicken breasts, light Italian bread, low-calorie cottage cheese, low-calorie cheddar cheese with rice crackers, four containers of Arizona Diet Green Tea, Minute Maid orange juice (that I'll divide into four parts to reduce sugar and calories), a frozen bag of calamari rings, a frozen bag of flounder fillets, a frozen bag of mixed vegetables, two frozen bags of Bird's-Eye spinach. In the produce section, I bought escarole, broccoli rabe, kale, swiss chard greens, fennel, one eggplant, two tomatoes, one cucumber, mango, blueberries, strawberries, three pears. I guess I'm going to starve the next few days but calorie count is low.

What is the moral of this story? Well, when we were

young, we ate anything that gave us pleasure with absolutely no guilt. I remember when I was first dating, we went to this Chinese restaurant and ordered a large (really large) plate of spare ribs. After we ate them, we ordered a second plate of spare ribs. Spare ribs (even one rib) are loaded with calories and we ate over 100 of the damn things.

Around middle age, I became a little more disciplined and held back on all the ice cream and pastries and pasta.

Now, in the golden years…we talk about diets. We talk about green tea. We talk about CQ10. We talk about greens. We talk about fresh fruit and fresh vegetables. We cook using little oil. We never fry anything. No bakery shops for us! And a juicy McDonald's burger is a cardinal sin.

Well, after shopping I decided to go to a local diner here in the area and get me a mozzarella grilled sandwich with bacon and cole slaw on the side with a dill pickle. Ordered a root beer float and walked out of the diner feeling good about myself.

For that cardinal sin, for the past month or so, I'm eating like a monk.

There, that's my contribution to fitness. The ancients were right! Modern science has now revealed that green tea contains powerful antioxidant and antimicrobial activity and other health-promoting properties. Discover the wisdom of the ancients and drink green tea for good health. EGCG.

Well, I agree with some of what he says, but everyone has their own opinion about fitness and I said this book would be different, so if the shoe fits, wear it. Thanks, Sal. Keep drinking that green tea, that's the only thing I agree with you on.

JIM DOYLE

JIM DOYLE has been a friend of my son Steven for many years. They played high school football together at Immaculate Conception in Montclair and then both went on to play varsity football at Ramapo College. They have remained good friends and Jim has really followed through on fitness. Here's his story.

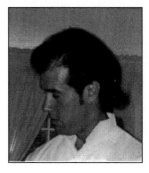

Jim Doyle

My workouts are geared towards health, fitness, and removing stress, and it helps me to stay sober (17 years). I have been a women's lacrosse official for eight years on the high school level and college game (Division 3). I run and sprint up and down a 120-yard field. I can usually do 30 to 40 lacrosse games from late March to early June. I work out at least four to five times a week, which always starts with 45 to 50 minutes of cardio. Treadmill – five-minute warm-up, 4% incline walk (4.0-4.2 speed); switch to walking backwards for five minutes, 4% incline; switch again to side lunges on treadmill for two minutes, both sides. It doesn't sound like much, but I am really loose after this and can go into a two to three mile run, or I do 110-yard and 220-yard sprints on Bucknell's track (outdoor-indoor). The sprints are to match my lacrosse running. For strength I do push-ups, pull-ups and dips two times a week. One day a week I still do free weights (only 20 to 25 minutes) and dumbbells for 8, 10 or 12 reps. During lacrosse season and summer months, I do circuit training on Hammer-Strength machines, rep out on any machine for 45 seconds and go to the next machine with about a 30-second break and rep out again on another machine. Example: Shoulder press for 45 seconds to almost fatigue or can't do another rep, rest 30 seconds and hit leg curls for 45 seconds, and then move to another machine. I do this for 20 minutes, and you will be shaking upon completion. I also do leg extensions and leg curls and leg press once a week for leg strength and balance workout. I do squats with a medicine ball against my back and on any wall: 10 to 12 reps, 3/4 squat down and ball rolls up-down your back. You can use dumbbells to increase weights.

I am a strong believer in walking and getting outside and getting fresh air. Polly (my wife) and I just walked today for one hour, and on my off day or light workout day I will walk 45 to 60 minutes. I bike ride in the spring, summer and fall. Diet is huge. I do protein drinks, oatmeal, yogurts, meats, salads, almonds, fruits, veggies. I am 210 lbs. on my 6'2" frame, and that is 10 lbs. under my senior high school year weight when I played football. While playing college football, my weight was 270 pounds. I am committed to staying fit.

Thanks, Jim. I remember when you were 270 pounds in college and playing tackle. Not too many people could move you. You have trimmed yourself down to a very healthy weight and your program sounds very healthy. Keep it up.

AUNT MARGARET

AN INTERVIEW WITH MY AUNT MARGARET

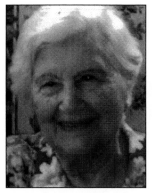

Aunt Margaret

It was one of those days when softball had to take "second base" and the rain wouldn't stop that I had an interview with one of my fittest seniors, who will be 100 years old in November of 2008. Although in a wheelchair, she's a still-going-strong powerhouse, despite not being able to hear as well as she would like...but sharp as ever.

Margaret Farano smiles as I ask my first question. "Aunt Margaret, what do you attribute your long healthy life to?" Looking directly at me with a twinkle in her eye and tears starting to dwell on her beautiful face, she says, "I attribute my longevity to having a very happy attitude all my life. And I did a lot of walking and was very active, never overeating...having five small meals a day, thoroughly chewing my food...and I still have my original teeth [she shows them to me], which allows me to eat whatever I want."

I look at a woman with a beautiful complexion no plastic surgeon could create and would marvel at her age. Both of her parents lived to be in their late nineties, so I guess genes do play a part in longevity, and I sure wish I had her teeth.

I will certainly be at her centennial celebration. After all, Ann Margaret Farano is my favorite aunt.

This next guy has been playing softball with me for many years and is probably the best center fielder in the league – you have to be in good shape to run like he does. Let's hear it from SAL GAMBINO (not from the publicized Gambino family).

SAL GAMBINO

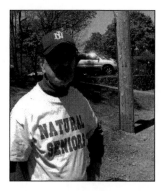

Sal Gambino

When I was young, ages about eleven to seventeen, I was restricted by my very strict father to play any sports, but because I loved sports so much, I would sneak away from my family's poultry market where I had to work. My father caught me doing this one time and really gave me some beating, and of course I had to go back to work. After I was drafted into the military, things really changed. I thought I was on vacation while everybody else was complaining. I joined the military softball team and touch football team, where we won both championships in 1955. That's basically how I started my sports career. After my discharge I worked for Eastern Airlines and regularly played basketball and softball for the airline's teams.

As far as diet goes, I start my day with a very light breakfast (usually cornflakes and bananas), green salad in the afternoon and a heavy dinner with a homemade glass of wine. Presently I have a mini gym at home where I have some equipment such as: bench, weights, trampoline, big ball, stationary bike, etc. I work out at least an hour a day or whenever I feel like doing it... I jog and run every night in the park or in the oval for thirty minutes.

I feel that two big factors that keep me healthy are never having smoked and being relaxed (very little stress), and of course being so active playing basketball, softball and running. I have been the same weight for over fifty years. I always drink plenty of water and eat plenty of fruits. I'm now 74, still expecting to play another ten years (at least). This is my simple secret to make me strong and healthy. Thanks, Tony, and I hope some of my suggestions can assist other people in their quest for a healthy and long life. Good luck, Tony – I hear your next book will be a novel. I can't wait to read it.

—Your buddy, Sal

PEGGY GOODMAN

PEGGY GOODMAN-ESTEY, at age 88, although now confined to a wheelchair, is still very fit. But she was a professional dancer, and I haven't seen too many fat dancers, have you? Let's hear the Peggy Goodman-Estey story.

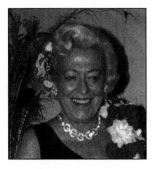

Peggy Goodman

It isn't easy being me, as I have been here on this earth as a dancer in body, heart, mind and soul for 88 years and I can't seem to get it straight that I'm supposed to stop. Not so. I won't give up, I can't give up, and I will dance until the day I die – well, almost.

Growing up in Montclair in the 1920's, theater was everything, especially the Montclair Operetta Club and the Montclair Dramatic Club. It seemed that all the boys and girls tap-danced, one better than the other. I don't know how I got the solos and the leads, but I did, and the joy of the Great American Songbook ruled the world. After graduating from Montclair High School, I became a Rockette at Radio City Music Hall and never looked back.

Fitness was a part of everyone's life, with the Great Depression keeping the pocketbook strings tighter than a drum. The fact that I married a man who went straight off to war in Europe kept me focused and dancing and eating correctly.

Over the years I invented something called Kinder Gym, which was teaching small children how to be agile and fit. This was long before organized gymnastics in America and, living in the shore area, I started off teaching at the local library.

For me, at the grand old age of 88, I continue to eat small meals throughout the day; never drink coffee; and dance whenever I can, especially sitting in my wheelchair and tapping my cane.

Thank you, Tony, for including me as the years flew away just remembering to always stay active in mind and body. You want to be fit? Just keep on dancing.

—Peggy Lake Goodman-Estey

Thanks, Peggy. It's people like you who give us an incentive to do something that we love, and dancing is certainly a FIT choice.

BARBARA GREICO

BARBARA GRIECO, the author of The Medical Notebook and retired physical education teacher, had this to say about staying fit.

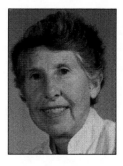

Barbara Greico

I believe that staying in shape involves three things. The first is a positive optimistic attitude towards life, which should be a firm belief in God. Why? Because when sadness or ill-fortune enters your life, and it will, we can put our trust in God to carry us through. An unhappy resentful person will not have the desire to stay in shape.

Secondly, a good diet is essential. A poor diet and emotional upheaval often lead to ill-health. I take supplements and buy organic food to compensate for our overuse of pesticides and chemical fertilizers on our farms. It is therefore difficult for a sick person to stay in shape.

Thirdly, regular aerobic exercise, outdoors in the sunlight, is absolutely necessary. I hike or walk, swim and folk dance. At age 76, with two total hip replacements, I had to give up tennis. However, I thank God for what I'm still able to do.

Thanks, Barbara, great attitude.

ROLF HABERMANN

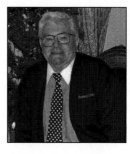

Rolf Habermann

My friend ROLF HABERMANN, at age 80, is still working every day and in pretty good condition, but when he was a young boy and in the "Hitler Youth" group, he was in excellent condition. He was, in fact, forced to be in excellent shape at the early age of ten, as it was mandatory in Germany to be a member of the Hitler Youth movement. Rolf has even written a book about it (Memory Of A Hitler Youth) and now, at the age of 80, the dictated habits of his youth fare him well as he continues to get up to go to work every day...with a smile. His habits have changed considerably but he hasn't forgotten the days when he had to get up before dawn in the dense fog of the seaport of Danzig on the Baltic Sea and, at certain times, run around an entire lake and then do very strenuous exercises with the rest of the boys.

No longer does he do those strenuous exercises, but he thinks nothing of constructing a three-story scaffold and still fearlessly climbing up when he builds another fireplace as the owner of Master Design Fireplaces...with over 400 fireplaces under his belt, fitness continues to dominate his vision. Rolf has workers doing a lot of the manual labor, but at age 80 he still works long hours and is on the job daily; he attributes this ability to his early exposure to the mantra taught when he was a pubescent boy. He has slackened somewhat on his diet and his weight is a little more than it should be, but he has never forgotten those days when he was a proud and healthy boy of the Hitler Youth. But let's *hear from Rolf.*

To me fitness is a very big part of character, determination and integrity with your own soul and is a discipline to your mind.

I say this because when I was barely ten years of age, living in Germany, I had to join the youth movement where sport and fitness was a very important part of your life...not just in school but in groups and camps within the youth movement. Consequently, this thinking process allowed fitness to synchronize with my character, and when I was in groups with other boys and girls, I wanted to look and do my best because I knew, at the end of the month, I would receive a medal to add to my collection and wear proudly on my uniform. There were three things which we had to live by and were brought up to be and continually emphasized: "You have to be as supple as leather, hard as Krupp steel and quick as a greyhound" – and those guidelines are still in my mind today at eighty years of age.

Some mornings I would want to lie in bed and sleep another hour and stay at home; however, it was branded in my brain, especially before a sports festival, where we had to warm up in the cold winter, spring, summer and fall by running two miles around a lake. We did not have softball, baseball or football but we did have soccer, and because I was so fast, in one scrimmage I was the fastest in the 60-meter even though my leg was wrapped with a slight sprain and the cloth was flying. Every achievement you were involved in, you had to look good with your classmates, your neighborhood and your town.

Today, when I step up on a train or get off of a plane, I always have the discipline to be fit and to avoid an accident. I may be a bit overweight but my kind of fitness has never been about weight lifting or going to the gym or even massaging my muscles to look good. Oh no, I still carry that little boy in me; that's why you have that image of the so-called "master race." But don't underestimate the reality that I am now a proud American today and I salute the boys who were fit to storm the beaches of Normandy...

That's enough of my explanation of fitness because my friend, Tony Naturale, the former police lieutenant and now an author, exemplifies what a true athlete is just by caring enough to document all of us.

Wow, thanks, Rolf, my AMERICAN FRIEND.

You certainly should give people an incentive to stay fit. And thank you for thinking to bring the AMERICAN FLAG to our SENOR OLYMPICS SOFTBALL TEAM (2005) when you were our team photographer and mascot in Pittsburgh and we won the Bronze Medal.

DONNA ROMAN HERNANDEZ

DONNA ROMAN HERNANDEZ's story could be a movie. Actually she is a producer and writer who has produced three films.

She was born and raised in Newark, New Jersey, and just recently retired as a captain from the Caldwell Police Department after serving 26 years in law enforcement. She was the recipient of the 2006 Garden State Woman of the Year in Government Award, and in 2007 was a Jefferson Award honoree for community service in New Jersey.

Donna is a multi-award-winning independent film director, producer, composer and orator. Currently, she is the Domestic Violence Response Team Coordinator for Babyland Family Services in Newark. Additionally, Donna is a Domestic Violence Trainer with the New Jersey Division of Criminal Justice, Office of the Attorney General.

When I saw Donna come through the door for our interview, I saw a person ready to greet life. Before we said our first "hello" I knew she was a cop, in spite of her fashionable jean jacket and dark sunglasses, as she circled the room and recognized me immediately without an introduction (cops can spot another cop a mile away).

I am eager to interview her as she has emerged as one of the most in-demand and versatile cops, comfortable as a speaker on a panel about "The Ultimate Betrayal: A Survivor's Journey," which is her true story of a "woman in blue" who lived her life under the shadows of family violence and who was haunted by the memories of an abusive father.

Donna has the energy of a five-man band playing all night long. Since she retired from the police force, Donna has embodied the adage that discretion is the better part of valor, lecturing on the perils of domestic violence to the public primarily through her films. She stated:

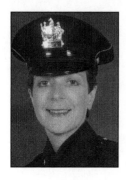

Donna Hernandez

I try to be balanced; nothing in this life is black or white. I've just turned fifty and I want to stay in good physical health. I work out in the gym with my personal trainer three times a week and also work out every day on my own, doing one hour of circuit training, aerobic walking with weights, and salsa dancing on the weekends in New York City. When I wake up I am filled with energy, and when I go to sleep I am filled with energy...good health is a state of mind and is the key to staying fit.

My eating habits consist of at least five meals a day every three hours, but small portions; I continually watch my fat and salt intake with absolutely no fried foods, no coffee or liquor. I'm into all sorts of spices, antioxidants, garlic, ginger, basil, oregano, sage, turmeric on all my vegetables. I boil low-fat meat after I have marinated it in lots of lemon juice to break up the fat and tenderize the meat.

My husband, Gerardo, sadly had a post-traumatic brain injury which was, at first, devastating as he had been a professional wrestler for the country of Cuba, so to continue good health for both of us, we keep a very strict diet. I have found that diet is the key for maximum health benefits, and we eat nutritionally healthy foods together. By the way, Gerardo trains three hours every day but we do not work out together.

Boy, Donna, I've let my readers know how active I and some of my fellow athletes are, but I believe you have surpassed many of us...and are still going strong. I am honored to include such an accomplished and focused woman. Your strong and dedicated commitment, not just for health but for life itself, continues through your films, which give hope and a better world to live in. God bless you.

ED HOFF

ED HOFF has been playing ball with me for many years. As the father of five daughters, he must be in shape. Let's hear it, Ed.

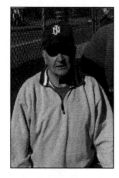

Ed Hoff

I have been physically active all my life. As a 12-year-old, my summer job was as a laborer on our new home that my father and grandfather were building. The job included mixing cement, setting blocks, handling lumber, plywood, and shingles. In school I played football, basketball, baseball and track, and golf on the outside. I always had a part-time job and as a senior I worked in a lumberyard. During college and after army service, I worked in lumberyards and a factory. After college I worked for a lumberyard chain, became manager, but was still humping sheetrock, plywood, and cement on a daily basis.

I married in 1961 and two years later took a job as a salesman on the road. My physical work then became remodeling the house and some softball. In 1972 we started a wholesale millwork business. I unloaded freight cars, sold moldings, loaded the truck and delivered the products for two years before hiring our first employee. I kept that pace for thirty years while growing the business, which we eventually sold in 2001.

In the early 1990's, I started softball in the 50-and-over league. When I retired, I started playing in the 60-and-over leagues on Saturday, Tuesday and Thursday.

I have also enjoyed playing basketball three days a

week on Mondays, Wednesdays and Fridays. In the winter months I alternate between basketball and the "Y" at 5:30 a.m. On softball days I usually go to the "Y" before a game.

As far as my diet goes, I have made some significant changes. One thing will never change, though, and that is Wednesday night is spaghetti night. In the mornings now I have a substantial breakfast. Usually it consists of orange juice, cereal, fresh fruit and coffee. Lunch is usually a large salad with olive oil dressing. At 4 p.m. each day I make popcorn and Crystal Lite as I watch [Neil] Cavuto. Dinner is whatever Peg prepares, and I usually finish my meal. I don't use much salt and pepper, but have become a salsa junkie. I had been a daily ice cream fan until I was diagnosed with type 2 diabetes. I have cut back on the ice cream, rarely eat desserts, and with the medication seem to have the diabetes under control.

In 2006 I started preparing for the Senior Olympics and lost 25 pounds via strenuous exercise and diet, and have managed to keep most of the weight off. I changed my eating habits, but still very much enjoy vodka martinis, Manhattans and good old beer.

I think the biggest incentive I have is to be with other men about my age who have the same love of sports as I do. I would much rather play two or three hours of softball amid the kibitzing of 20 to 25 men than to play five hours of golf in a reserved environment while riding around in a cart. I have met many bright, articulate, funny, and kind men over the years. I marvel at the accomplishments of many in the business and athletic world. We have all found our field of dreams.

I have been very fortunate to have my loving wife Peggy for the last 46 years and to be the proud father of five daughters and one son, and grandfather of five granddaughters and four grandsons. I want to see the young people grow, graduate, marry and become parents, and that is good enough reason for staying fit. I had been a three-pack-a-day smoker for many years, even after my dad died at 57 from emphysema and heart problems. He also was a diabetic, had glaucoma and other illnesses. My mom died at ninety and hopefully I have her genes. My only sibling, my brother Ray, died at 59. I am 71 and probably as fit as I was at fifty. God has been very good to me.

I marvel at the accomplishments of the men who were policemen, firemen, military retirees, teachers, blue-collar workers and businessmen who were outstanding athletes in years past and are still playing on their "field of dreams."

Ed, I have watched you play ball for the past ten years now and you're right, GOD HAS BEEN GOOD TO YOU. He has been good to all of us "oldsters" playing this boys' game at our age. It has been a pleasure to play with such an accomplished person and I know you will be around to see your grandchildren grow up.

KATE HURLEY

My granddaughter, KATIE HURLEY, has a good concept on fitness. Let's hear it, Katie.

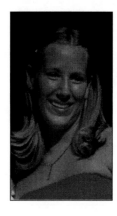

Kate Hurley

I'm a 22-year-old recent college graduate who's been playing sports since she could walk. The majority of my fitness workouts have come in the form of sports practices created by the variety of coaches I've had throughout the years and my own training I do between seasons. Playing soccer, basketball, track and rugby, I've learned a lot about working out. For instance, each sport requires different needs from your body – whether that's endurance for soccer or the ability to continually get up and down in rugby.

For athletes, training needs to be specifically oriented toward whatever demands the game/match/event puts on one's body. Overall, there are a million and one different ways to work out, but it's imperative that you create workouts that will help you accomplish your personal goals.

I do my best to lead a very healthy lifestyle and I believe that I have all the knowledge necessary to be a so-called "health nut," as my grandfather would put it. My biggest obstacle lies in my willpower to eat as healthy as I know I should be. During my time at the University of Massachusetts, Amherst, I struggled with eating. College for so many students is a whirlwind of beer, parties, lots of fried foods, and I suppose on occasion a bit of class and studying. I know how important eating well is, but eating less healthy is often cheaper, easier, and faster. (I'm not talking about fast food restaurants but supermarkets like Whole Foods versus your average grocery store.) Since college ended, I've been working much harder to overcome the fear of eating well so I can achieve the utmost of healthy lifestyles.

In conclusion, here are a few key elements I believe and live by in order to maintain a healthy fit lifestyle (whether you're trying to lose weight, maintain, or improve your fitness). First, no matter how hard and long you spend working out, none of it matters if you're not eating correctly. Second, to be successful in a routine, one must set smaller achievable goals as opposed to one nearly unreachable high goal. This will make it easier to stick to the routine. Third, change up your routine, because the body adjusts to workouts and that is when you hit plateaus. Fourth, any workout is better than no workout at all – it's important to pick an exercise you're actually going to do. Finally, don't starve yourself or get caught up in fad diets.

In order to lose weight and keep it off, you need to learn how to eat right while making positive lifestyle changes.

Wow, Katie, for a young lady you certainly seem to be wise in the fitness equation. If you follow your advice, you will certainly be in better shape than your Poppop.

DR. MICHAEL KELLY

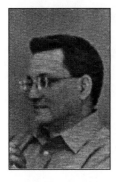

Dr. Michael Kelly

Now here's a person we should all listen to: Doctor MICHAEL KELLY, a friend of mine and also my orthopedic doctor, who has many skills. He is the assistant chief ringside physician for the New Jersey State Athletic Control Board. He is also an accomplished expert in the martial arts and holds multiple black belts. He not only is teaching sports medicine, but through his books and periodicals that he has published, he is teaching patients, athletes and caregivers the basics of sports medicine in a select field of sports for which he has a passion, namely martial arts.

He has been involved in martial arts since he was a child and has been inducted into the Universal Martial Arts Hall of Fame. Additionally, he has authored and published the books *Death Touch, the Science Behind the Legend of Dim-Mak* and just recently *Fight Medicine*. These are only some of the qualifications of this very talented doctor.

To quote Doctor Kelly, "My general advice to my patients about exercise is to stay active, injury free, and train in moderation. You do not have to train like a professional athlete to remain in good health. The key, I believe, is moderation and to have fun. Keep it simple and interesting. Motion is more important than method, and of course maintain a good diet. Good luck."

Thanks, Doc, for your words of wisdom.

GENE KELLY

This next person married Doctor Kelly's brother, Gene. No, not the Hollywood famed Gene Kelly, but still someone who can cut a rug and give an old softshoe. But Maddie Kelly is a professional dancer and choreographer and, after looking at the promo and all the Broadway memorabilia hanging in the sunny salon of their home, I said to myself, "Boy, is she in shape." I knew it was not going to be easy to track her down, but as hubby is Maddie's number-one fan, I decided to give GENE KELLY an ear and let him toot her horn before she arrived for the interview. (By the way, most of my friends call me Natch.)

Tony, let me give you a few good, full and easy-on-the-draw facts about my beautiful wife, as she is all too humble, a mere mite at 5'3" and 100 pounds of kryptonite and gamma rays of sheer delight – with no body fat, mind you. And are you ready for this, Natch? The consistent winner of the "All Broadway Yearly (Gag) Award," my wife: Madeleine Ehlert Kelly – Maddie is known for "What a body!" or "The best butt on Broadway"!

If you were to look at Maddie's athletic ability alone, it would never touch her creative genius, as she has a mathematical brain. Why, Chita Rivera, the explosive and exciting dancer who rocketed to stardom in "West Side Story" over fifty years ago, and star of "A Dancer's Life," considers herself to be Maddie's stepmother. So does the beautiful Graciela Daniel, who was in the original cast of "Chicago" – she feels the same way. Chita had her as the dance captain/swing in "A Dancer's Life" and Graciela had her as the ensemble/stunt specialty creator for "Annie Get Your Gun," also working with Bernadette Peters.

Thanks, Gene. And look who's here, straight from the Big Apple. Let's hear the MADELEINE KELLY story.

MADELEINE KELLY

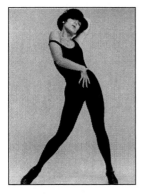

Madeleine Kelly

I'm coming at you like a swirling dervish because this is who I am! God danced the day I was born and somehow, by osmosis, and through the gentle whisperings in my ear from my daddy and the tunes played on the radio Mommy sang, I wiggled my toes and was a miniature Ginger Rogers straight out of my diapers. I walked early, talked early and started taking dancing lessons early

As one of three sisters, we seemed to be "Rockettes" before we even came down from Rhode Island to see the bright lights of the Big Apple. But somehow I have to slow down to let you know what it is that keeps me fit. For all too many wonderful years I have been assisting with the creation of Broadway shows and will be doing "Pal Joey" for Broadway with Patty Lupone in the fall, as well as hiring for Disney cruises – keeps me more than busy. I was the director and associate director and choreographer for "A Dancer's Life" as well as Lincoln Center. Plus I am a very happily married woman, married to Gene Kelly (no relation to that Hollywood dancing star). However, at our wedding we had seven brides for seven sisters in our wedding party and the bridesmaids all did a "high kick," as did my groom.

It is mandatory that I stay fit and it is second nature to me. We live in an old farmhouse with lots of land in Essex Fells. I cut the grass with an electric mower and wear headphones, which allows me to design and create routines for my shows, losing all sense of time and, before I know it, the lawn is done and another new dance routine is born.

As a gift to myself I buy fresh flowers every week as well as fresh fruit, but I don't stop there. I cut the fruit up and put it in little baggies daily and will snack on it throughout the day. There are also homemade oatmeal cookies with dates, nuts and chopped fruits – but only a few to each bag. My husband Gene is a gourmet chef, for us, and is continually concocting exquisite marinades with fresh herbs from my garden for fish, veal and chicken.

We have a beautiful Doberman pinscher called "Lacey" who needs a lot of exercise, hence I take her to a nearby park for "socialization" in the morning and she runs after balls thrown into the woods by either Gene or myself; depending on how up and at 'em we are is who takes her for her morning run and who takes the afternoon run. We both belong to a gym but go when it is convenient for our schedules.

As I take the bus into Manhattan, I am usually running to catch the bus in or to catch the bus home. I am your perpetual woman in motion so I burn a lot of calories and have never had a weight problem. Yogurt is a Godsend and I sometimes, for extra energy, put oatmeal in it. My secret I think has been that I always make sure I have a protein, carbohydrate and a complex carbohydrate, and I eat little meals throughout the day.

Coming from a large family and having Dr. Michael Kelly as my brother-in-law inspired me to share my feelings on staying fit. He is a sports doctor, an author and someone who is very interested in seeing that the whole family stays fit. I knew I had to take the time to talk to Natch. Why? Because I believe he cares.

Wow, Maddie, I certainly do care and I am honored to have someone so fit and with your credentials be a part of my book. Keep it up and GIVE MY REGARDS TO OLE BROADWAY.

BILL KENNEDY

BILL KENNEDY was a Newark News sports reporter whom I played softball with many years ago, and at age 67 he still manages to be very active. Here's his story straight from the reporter's mouth.

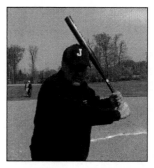
Bill Kennedy

Bill Kennedy (me) of Glen Ridge, NJ, is able to continue to play and enjoy three sports: four-wall handball, slow-pitch softball and golf.

How is that possible for a man of that age who is overweight? Genes are the main reason. His father, William C. Kennedy Sr., is 95 and in very good health. He had cataract surgery two years ago, and that was the first time he ever had stayed in a hospital overnight. Hernia surgery was done on him probably years ago, but other than that, the senior Kennedy has been almost a medical marvel. His mother died at age 88. She was a smoker until 85, or she probably would have lived longer.

So longevity is in Bill Jr.'s genes. Another longevity ingredient (at least in my opinion) is swimming. He was raised swimming in Lake Kanawaukee, which is in Harriman Park in New York State near Tuxedo. From there he went to boys' camp during the summers and became a very good swimmer and diver – mostly for the Montclair YMCA swim team. Swimming tends to elongate muscles, and over the years that certainly has helped Kennedy's athletic pursuits.

Kennedy played basketball and baseball through high school and college. When he was 25, Kennedy was playing basketball in three leagues and fast-pitch softball in two. There was a gap between seasons – March to May. It was then that former Boston College and NFL guard Bill Byrne introduced Kennedy to four-wall handball at the Montclair YMCA.

That sport also kept Kennedy fit and young. At age 67, he is playing handball three times a week at Classic in Fairfield, NJ, and that helps to keep the motor running. Kennedy became a very good age group handball player. He won some open tournaments in doubles, but after turning forty, he won a state and regional singles championship, a national doubles championship, and numerous state and regional doubles titles in his age group.

Heavier and slower now, the body wears down much more quickly than it did when Kennedy was in his thirties playing handball almost every day. But the fact that he can do it three times a week, and play in weekend tournaments, is a testament to his biggest sport. And make no mistake about it. Handball keeps Kennedy sharp for softball, and he has learned how to play handball one day and golf the next without being terrible on the golf course. That once was a huge problem. The two sports did not mix at all.

Why is this important to Kennedy? "I'd have to say that the worst thing that could happen to me physically at this stage of my life would be to start slowing down. If I play less or stop playing completely, the aging process is going to speed up. I've seen this in many of my contemporaries. Hey, it will happen soon enough. The body will make me quit. But I am not giving in easily."

What has been accomplished by the Kennedy body, if you consider any of this to be noteworthy, has been done mostly through activity. He used to run, but in his forties, he developed hip and back problems, so he stopped. He does some light weight training with 20-pound dumbbells. But mostly it is the competition which keeps him going.

Handball is No. 1. Walking eighteen holes is No. 2. Softball is No. 3, but that has slowed down almost to a halt in the last few years. Tony Naturale is trying to get Kennedy back to softball. That could happen.

You also have to factor in good luck. Kennedy's handball regimen has included a Wednesday noon game of doubles for almost thirty years. Kennedy and his twenty-year partner, Tom Lynch, 66, would play the team of two of three men – Ed Kaliner, 66, Mike Meltzer, 61, and Ken Smolack, 61. Lynch and Kaliner have had a hip replacement. Meltzer has had both hips replaced. Smolack has had a knee replacement. Kennedy, the oldest member of the group, has managed to survive without surgical replacements. His only surgery has been a double hernia in 2000. And he takes no meds. None. That is pure luck.

No magic formula is involved with Bill Kennedy. He drinks beer and enjoys cocktails.

This summer, Kennedy and his wife, Kathy, have been at their vacation home on Thompson Lake in Otisfield, Maine. That involves a lot of swimming, a lot of walking on the golf course, a lot of work around the place, which adds up to a lot of fresh Maine air. Five months have been spent there. Will that result is anything positive physically for Kennedy? Time will tell.

He said, "Whatever I have is the product of good genes and Anheuser Busch."

Bill, you underestimate yourself. Yes, good genes play a part, but you have been very active throughout your years and that has allowed you to be in the shape you are in. Wow, playing handball, that alone is enough activity to keep you in shape. Now let's throw in a little softball, a little less beer, and you can be an "Adonis." See you on the ball field.

BILL KOSKY

The following is from my good friend and fellow ball player BILL KOSKY. Go, Bill.

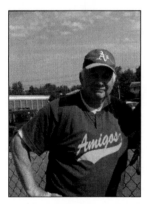
Bill Kosky

Like my longtime friend "Natch," I always felt good health was a priority in active living. As a youngster I participated in athletics as a means of staying in good shape, and softball, basketball and tennis kept me busy. Oh! I forget to mention the martial arts. I achieved the black belt in 1966. In 2003 and 2005, along with "Natch," I played in the national Senior Olympics in the softball tournament. Today at 74 years of age, my activities still include softball, golf and the martial arts. I have found the key to good health: commitment. I instruct at the Oak Ridge Martial Arts Academy three times a week. We have a special program for active adults (45 years and older) in which we emphasize stretching, to me the most important low-impact exercise, and self-defense techniques.

"Natch," thank you for the opportunity to be a part of your latest book.

—*Bill*

Thanks, Bill, see you on the ball field.

BOB KRUSE

I just met BOB KRUSE this year playing in the over-60 softball league and he's quite a ball player. Let's let him tell you his story (and he's not from Brooklyn).

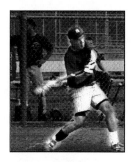

Bob Kruse

Since I was young boy, I loved playing any kind of ball. I lived in Union City, NJ, and there were not many available fields to use, so consequently I played a lot of stickball, football and basketball in either the street or the neighborhood school yard.

When I was ten or eleven years old, I tried out for the local Little League teams, but I was not selected to play. When I was in high school, I tried out for baseball and basketball my first two years and was not selected to play either. Since I was rejected from organized school ball, I still played in various pickup games in the neighborhood. I finally did get selected to play on a local Babe Ruth team when I was fifteen. It was very exciting to me. After high school, I went to work in NYC for an insurance company. There I was able to play intra-department softball and basketball games which were organized.

I was married in my early twenties, and at that time, through work in NJ, I was able to play on the company fast pitch (windmill) softball. But in my thirties I stopped playing altogether for about five or six years while my kids were growing up, and I was involved in their activities. Then when I was about forty, my son was now starting to play in a local softball league and I joined him on his team. It was a wonderful experience playing together, which we did for about ten years. Around that time my son stopped playing, but I continued playing in numerous leagues. I played in all age categories until I was around sixty, and then I decided that I needed to stick to playing with guys around my own age. For the past ten years, I have averaged playing in over 100 games each year. In 2007, I played in 135 games. This is considerable for living in the Northeast. It is also a huge difference from the initial league I started playing in with my son, which only played a thirteen-game season (once weekly). The point of providing all this background is to give the reader a feel for how much I love to play softball. As a normal practice, I have traveled over an hour to get to games in some of my leagues. During the season, I play in five leagues.

When I was 59 years old, I got up one morning for work, and stumbled and fell down while getting out of bed. My wife asked if I was okay, and naturally I told her yes, and that I just slipped getting up. The fact of the matter was that I was very dizzy. Being the "smart" person I am, I proceeded downstairs to get ready for work. First I let the dog out, and then was fixing the dog food, when the next thing I knew I was lying on the kitchen floor, with the dog licking my face. I had passed out. My wife heard me fall, and called 911. I was taken to the hospital, and it was found that my heart had gone into arterial fibrillation, and my heart rate had gone so low, it caused me to pass out. As I understand, a-fib is an abnormality in which some of the electrical impulses of the heart shut down. The main danger, besides passing out, is that while in this state, blood clots could develop and get thrown off to various parts of your body. Later that same day, my heart rhythms returned to normal on its own. However, my doctor then put me on regular dosages of blood thinners to minimize any blood clotting should this happen again.

Over the next few years, it did reoccur, but now my heart had to be "shocked" back to normal rhythm each time. In early 2004, one month after I retired, it happened again. This time my doctor advised me that I needed a pacemaker. I was very apprehensive about getting this foreign object implanted in my body. I thought that it would debilitate me from all my softball activities. My doctor assured me that it would not. He told me that I only had to take things easy for 8-10 weeks after the surgery, and that then I could return to do whatever I wanted to do. I was still apprehensive as I awaited the time to go by until I could play.

Prior to playing again, both my wife and I were concerned that since I pitch in most games I play in, and that through the years, I am always getting balls hit off my body, that we needed to come up with something to protect the area where my pacemaker is. We investigated various sources, but didn't come up with an answer. Then my wife came up with the idea that we make something ourselves. I bought a knee pad, elastic material, and Velcro. We then went to a shoemaker in Morristown, and asked if he could work with us in creating this protection. My wife directed him as to how to measure it, where to cut, and where to sew it together, and add the Velcro. The result was what seems like a one-of-a-kind padding which I have been wearing to protect my pacemaker when I pitch. Fortunately, since wearing it, I have never had a ball hit off of it. I still do get dings to other parts of my body though.

Well, now I am 67 years old and playing and enjoying playing softball more than ever. In fact this year, I was asked to join a softball team made of NJ Seniors in the 65-70 age bracket, which went to the Senior Olympics in Louisville, Kentucky. We played eight games in three days, and won a Gold Medal for our age group for the State of New Jersey. It was a truly wonderful experience. In addition, I belong to the YMCA in Morristown. I work out there three times a week, using the treadmill and light weights.

Bob, you have made a great comeback since your operation and have become one of the best ball players in our seniors league. I wish you were on my team. Good luck and I'll see you on the ball field.

NANCY LAGIA

GARY LAGIA, at age sixty, is one of our younger ball players. He, in fact, plays in an over-30 league and if you saw him play, you would think he is around that age. Let's hear what keeps you in shape, Gary, and how you can hit that ball like a young man... but before we hear from Gary, his wife NANCY has a few words to say about him. Go, Nancy.

As his wife of 38 years, I have witnessed how consistent and disciplined he is in his everyday habits. He eats low fat and drinks wine with his evening meal.

His stamina is never-ending and I tease him about "leaving his body to science." In our next life, I want his body and he can have mine. It's great for him, but being married to such an "Eveready battery" sure wears me out.

But most important is his positive "can do" mental attitude. Fielding errors, bad at-bats, or a poor golf shot results in a challenge to improve on the next opportunity. Mental toughness and determination work in conjunction with his fitness.

His optimistic outlook on life contributes to a peaceful mind. He sleeps well and lives large. That is why I think that man will be playing ball till he's 100!!!

Thank you, Tony, for allowing me to give some input on Gary's fitness.

—Nancy Lagia, Gary's wife

Okay, GARY, now it's your turn.

GARY LAGIA

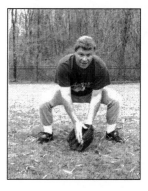

Gary Lagia

I just turned sixty in July 2007 so I've got a way to go to get to your level of conditioning at 76 years young, Tony, but I plan on staying in shape for many years to come.

I've always been active, playing baseball/softball (my first love), basketball, football, tennis and golf growing up. I've played organized softball since college (intramural softball was huge). In later years, I've been on two to three leagues every season, playing at least 60 or 70 games every year. I spent about 25 years playing in both the modified fast pitch and 6-12' arc leagues. I had a lot of fun and made a lot of good friends.

When I turned 35, the town of Montville, New Jersey started a very competitive over-30 league. I still play in the league to this day, serving as commissioner for the past twenty years. I enjoy competing against players 25 years younger than I. I've actually been hitting the ball better over the past couple of years than when I was much younger: had consecutive game hitting streaks of 25 and 26 games over the last two seasons. (Don't worry – Joe D's record is safe!) Since I'm the oldest player in the league, I'm affectionately known as the "ageless wonder."

My real fitness story develops around having a lot of energy and having a fairly high cholesterol level – thanks to my parents (who both passed away in their mid 60's). When I was about 35, I discovered that the high level of LDL (bad cholesterol) was at a point where diet and exercise alone weren't going to do the job, so I started on the medication route. Of course, diet and exercise would also have to be a part of my life if I wanted to be at the grandkids' weddings. I had always watched what I ate anyway (well, sort of), but decided to really change my eating habits, eliminating as much fat and cholesterol from my diet as possible. Red meat became only an occasional treat; I practically live on chicken, broccoli and pasta. My family and friends kid me about bothering to look at a menu at restaurants, since I always wind up ordering some sort of chicken or pasta dish!

My weight has stayed at about 165 (170-175 in the winter) for the past 25 to 30 years.

Breakfast usually consists of cold cereal with skim-plus milk and a piece of fruit or, on weekends, a bagel with Smart Balance spread. Lunch during the week is a can of fat-free soup or a salad. Weekends I may go crazy and eat a sandwich!

I have a workout room in my basement where, fall and winter, I try to get about two to three hours in weekly – mostly treadmill, stretching and lifting weights (less weight, more reps).

During spring and summer I don't work out, since there are four to five softball games and a couple of rounds of golf each week.

My routine seems to work for me, since I've only missed one season of softball in the last forty years (herniated disc in 1984 at age 37).

I truly believe my consistent regimen of diet and exercise has kept me injury free all these years. I always stretch at home prior to a game and make sure I get to the field early enough to stretch again, run, throw and take a few swings just to loosen up. All too often I've seen players pull something or suffer some other kind of injury because they didn't warm up properly.

I hope the people reading this book will find this info useful.

Good luck with the book, Tony, and I'll see you on the ball field.

Thanks, Gary, and the way you play, I can see why you still play in the over-30 league. I'm glad you decided to play with us old guys too, and thank you, Nancy, for your input. See you (Gary) on the ball field. Sorry, Nancy, it's a men's league.

SUSAN FINNEY LEFAVE

As a proud graduate of Montclair High School, I am honored to have a fellow Montclair High School graduate, SUSAN FINNEY LEFAVE, as a part of my book. She has the unique distinction of being the first woman ever inducted into Montclair High School's Athletic Hall of Fame, joining such notables as Coach Clary Anderson, Coach Butch Fortunato, and Astronaut Edwin "Buzz" Aldrin, to name a few. Her dad, Howard Finney Jr., coached the Cobras Little League, and I was one of his first assistants who used to see this very young little girl (Sue) outrun many of the ball players. She went on to become quite an athlete and set many records in ice hockey and field hockey. I watched her progress throughout the years and it was inevitable that she should gain recognition by achieving such an amazing goal of getting into the Montclair High School Hall of Fame. Here's her story:

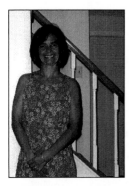

Susan Finney LeFave

When I left Montclair High School in 1986, I went to Princeton University, where I continued to excel in women's athletics, having played field hockey and women's ice hockey. In 1990, I graduated with a BA in Art History, and then two years later entered Boston College Graduate School, where I earned two master's degrees in Elementary and Special Education.

From Boston, I took a special education teaching position in Hawaii and taught there for four years. It was in Hawaii where I met my husband, Steve Lefave, through softball. I also played on a women's tennis team and paddled on a Hawaiian canoe team.

84

Steve and I married in 1998 and moved to New Orleans, where he was to begin a new tour as a Lieutenant for the United States Coast Guard. He has since retired after 23 years. I continued to teach in New Orleans for another three years. My son Tyler was born in 2000 and my daughter Lily was born in 2002.

During my athletic years, I never had to watch what I ate – until I went to college. In college I was not eating right, though I continued to play field hockey and women's ice hockey throughout my years at Princeton. I had never really liked the conditioning programs and weightlifting programs of college sports. I just wanted to play the sport. By the time I went to graduate school in 1994, I weighed 138 pounds! For a small-sized individual at 5'2", I knew some lifestyle changes were needed regarding my eating habits.

After college and graduate school, I started eating more protein foods like fish and chicken and cutting down on my starchy foods. I ate more veggies and started to cut down on my sugar intake. In Hawaii, I took up weight training with a professional body builder at the gym, using free weights instead of Nautilus machines to tone my body. I supplemented my workout with Hawaiian canoeing, tennis, and softball.

By the time I got married in 1998, I was down to what I weighed my senior year in high school, 108 lbs. I can proudly say that I still weigh 108 lbs. I have maintained a balanced diet and exercise routine. I work out at the gym up to four times a week, mixing a cardio workout of a Cybex machine, spinning classes, and kickboxing along with free weights and hammer strength machines. Though I do not currently play on an organized sports team, my children keep me very busy, especially my speedy five-year-old daughter, Lily!!!

Sue, you have had an amazing athletic career and I am honored to have such a notable athlete as part of my book. It sounds like Lily has your genes and your speed. Good luck.

WALTER MALY

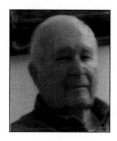

Walter Maly

WALTER MALY never exercised much in his early years while teaching as an elementary school teacher but started playing softball in his late fifties. I met Walt about 15 years ago and he was playing and managing the New Jersey Embers from West Orange. I only played two years with them but did go to the Senior Olympics with him. Walt is quite a pitcher and actually pitched a shut-out in the Olympics, which is quite a task in softball.

So why is Walt in this fitness book? Walt had a hip operation approximately two years ago and not long after, had to have a heart valve replaced. Since that has occurred, Walt has become a new person. He walks almost every day and hits the YMCA three times a week. At 5'10" and almost 220 pounds when he started, he is now trimmed down to 195. After consulting a nutritionist, his eating habits have changed drastically. His breakfast is mostly oatmeal with walnuts and raisins and bananas, and his lunch and dinner portions are much smaller. In between meals he will usually have fruit and will not eat anything after his evening meal. Walt said since he started the exercise program he feels much better, and at age eighty years young, looks forward to a long life. His physical activities have increased in his later years, and he is in much better shape since he has increased his activities.

Great, Walt, you are living proof that it's never too late to start a program. Keep it up and I know you will be pitching against me again very soon.

JACK MCGROATHY

The next person, one of my best ball players, has quite a story to tell. Let's hear from JACK McGROATHY, the former Essex County police officer. Go, Jack.

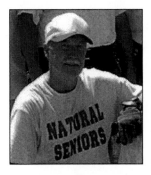

Jack MCGroathy

Competition is life's prescription for success. As in athletics, competitive spirit creates the human desire to drive one's genetic and developed capabilities to exceed their potential physical and psychological limits.

As a young boy being raised in a local suburb of Newark, New Jersey, it became apparent that athletics and competition would be an important part of that development. The organizational sports that were available at that time in the early fifties were the common sports of football, basketball and baseball. Engaging in these endeavors meant the development of strength and agility to perform at an adequate level. Family cohesion, spiritual stability and organizational sports provide a meaningful structure for a young person to develop into a productive adult. Sadly, I did not have this.

Organized sports became my initial introduction in an attempt to secure that potential. With that in mind, Little League baseball became a perfect start for that process. Learning the basic fundamentals, as in all sports, was challenging and a struggle, yet the need to perform better was a significantly strong driving factor that remains with me until this day.

Listening to and watching baseball's heroes of yesteryear, and wanting to be like them, was a force to be reckoned with for a young boy. Who didn't want to be in the enviable position of coming to the plate with two outs in the bottom of the ninth, the bases loaded and down one run? Hitting that home run that won the big one was every boy's dream. As in life, that is not always to be the resulting outcome. Failure is as much a part of the process of maturity as is success.

High school offered me additional opportunities to challenge myself in different athletic activities. Football built strength and agility, gymnastics created balance and coordination. When it came time to play baseball, I chose a different path of track and field. Being a mile runner produced endurance and stamina, and being a pole-vaulter combined both balance and strength.

After high school, my thoughts turned towards career choices. Not wanting to abandon my ardor for athletics and a desire to maintain strong personal character, I knew from my early years that my eventual choice would be in the line of law enforcement. In 1971, I was accepted into the Essex County Police Department. I shortly discovered that life in an urban police environment meant that not only could I combine my fondness for physical fitness with my career, but it became mandatory.

I was fortunate enough to escalate through the ranks and eventually earned the opportunity to become a training advisor and lead instructor in the physical training program at the Police Academy. This opportunity afforded me the chance to instill in the mindset of the recruits the significance and value of attaining and maintaining good physical condition. To reinforce and emphasize these principles, I found it necessary and important to not require the recruit officers to perform any physical tasks that I myself could not complete. This assignment enabled me to remain on the path of maintaining a personal physical fitness regimen.

After retirement from a very rewarding and successful career in law enforcement, I found the time to rekindle my fondness for America's favorite pastime. I began slowly, playing softball in a night league, but eventually expanded my playing to three leagues with a reintroduction to hardball and traveling tournament play. The skills learned long ago, although somewhat diminished, quickly resurfaced and my affection for the game of baseball promptly renewed.

My trek through life was nearly derailed by a diagnosis of esophageal cancer in 2004. As with all cancers, the prestage is always somewhat debatable. After a very successful operative procedure, the prognosis radically deteriorated when I dropped into a septic state. After falling into a coma lasting 11 days, the real struggle ensued to rehabilitate and strengthen an acutely weakened body. Recognizing the dilemma from a medical perspective, that only a fit condition permitted me to survive the initial procedure, the decision was obvious. The grueling effort, compounded with complications and setbacks, took a demanding ten months. Once again, my long dedication to a fitness ethic proved to be a major determining factor in my survival and my ability to return to the game I so loved. It took all of the learned and developed characteristics of life to triumph over the debilitating nature of the disease. This came from my deep spiritual stability, support of loved ones and a strong desire to survive.

Throughout my life, experiences in sports, my career as a police officer, and my near-fatal encounter with cancer have taught me many valuable lessons. One is that of integrity. Integrity is a personal character trait that no one can deprive you of; you can only surrender it. But first and foremost, faith, family and love are the true measures of life's success. Many times in one's life, it's the tribulations that breed faith, unify family and permit love to endure.

Maybe many of my life's efforts have not always eventuated as I would have liked, but in retrospect, my life's voyage has been one that I would not have wanted to live in any other way. Finally, nearing the autumn of my life, I really have become that little boy in the bottom of the ninth who hit the big one!

Jack, your inspirational story should motivate many people to be fit. If you were not in the physical condition you were in, I'm sure you wouldn't have come out as well as you have. Your present playing and your amazing acrobatic plays in both baseball and softball have been an inspiration to me and most of the players. I am honored to have you part of this book and part of my team. See you on the ball field.

TOMMY ANTHONY MELLINA

Well, I guess more than just a tree grew in Brooklyn. Here's another ball player who also grew up in Brooklyn. Go, TOMMY ANTHONY MELLINA (I like your middle name).

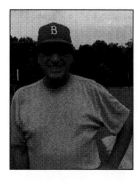

Tommy Anthony Mellina

There was no game of ball I did not play: stoop ball, baseball, handball, Chinese handball, softball, basketball, football, stickball, punchball, and boxball. These were games we played in Brooklyn. Never would a guy be seen carrying a tennis racquet or golf bag in my neighborhood. Brooklyn was too macho for those types of sports. The penalty would be ridicule or a beating!

As a teenager, I played baseball at the Brooklyn Parade Grounds, where players were constantly under the watchful eye of Major League scouts. My teen years were exciting times.

After I got married and was still living in Brooklyn, I played competitive basketball and softball. In the early 1970's I took a job in New Jersey and relocated my young family. Basketball and softball leagues continued to be a part of my life until 1976, when I accepted a position with a company that relocated me to Central Jersey. With an office in New York City and another one in New Jersey, and the demands of a new job, I had very little time for sports. However, after I finished working in my New Jersey office, I would do some running at the local high school track. I can look back on this time in my life as probably the only time I had, to myself, to stay in shape.

In 1980, I accepted an executive position at a major entertainment company in Manhattan and remained there until I retired in 1997. During that time, the extent of my staying in shape was getting on and off planes, driving to and from work in the city, and an occasional round of golf. Business lunches and dinners took their toll, so when I retired, I had to find a way to get back into shape. For a lot of people, getting in shape is not a priority. When I was much younger, my eating habits were not a high priority. However, in 1978, I did stop eating red meat of any kind as a result of talking to someone who introduced me to a book called *Survival Into the 21st Century*. Fortunately for me, too, I never started habits like smoking, drinking coffee, salting food, eating egg yolks or butter. I have the good fortune of having good family genes, along with being very concerned about eating certain types of food, ingredients in that food and food preparation.

With the exception of my grandmother, who died at the age of 86, all of my other elder relatives died after the age of 90, and most have lived to tell about it in great detail! My mother just celebrated her 90th birthday this spring (2007), and her memory of things that happened long ago is just as sharp as things that happened yesterday, as well as things that are still happening. She can flip from one subject to the next and not skip a beat! She is a devoted Mets fan and faithfully watches every game they play. In addition, she and I usually talk about the game from the day before, where she vividly recreates the successful (and unsuccessful) plays, including the do's and don'ts of managing a baseball team.

Constantly watching baseball games just might be the key to longevity!

After my retirement from the corporate world in 1997, I became the family handyman. I remodeled the kitchen and the rest of our vacation home in Florida, and I do all the maintenance work for our home in New Jersey. I also began to add moderate exercise to my daily routine and managed to play golf with more regularity. In 2003, my wife was speaking with our daughter's fifth grade teacher, and the subject of playing baseball came up. She casually mentioned that her husband regularly played baseball and that he was currently in Florida playing in a tournament.

As a result of that conversation, my life would change forever.

I was invited to work out and play ball with men who would soon become my best friends. I began a new baseball/softball career. I have been playing steadily in league tournaments with these guys, who are extremely dedicated to the game of baseball and who are in great shape. My search for an incentive to feel young, be healthy, exercise and work on staying in shape was over! I had found a comfortable place to be, physically and mentally. We all want the same thing: to have fun, to exercise and to be as healthy as possible for as long as possible.

Currently, I play softball four days a week (which translates into six games) and participate in baseball workouts, which take place on Thursday mornings. Because the level of my activities is extensive and intense, I take time to do isometrics and stretching exercises to keep from getting injured and to stay loose. I do not abuse my body by overdoing and have maintained a healthy weight of 192 lbs. on a 6'3" frame.

One regret is that I did not make friends with these guys sooner than 2003. The friendship and camaraderie are sincere, unconditional and as contagious as a mutual admiration society.

Having good friends is very important to good health. Many thanks to Tony (the Natural) for offering me an opportunity to contribute to his book. I only wish I could be as disciplined as he is. Good eating habits are as important as exercise.

Balance your approach to good health and remember what they say: "You are what you eat."

Thanks, Tom Anthony. As a fanatic Mets fan myself, I think I have to get together with your mom so we can discuss the Mets' problems. Maybe she should manage the Mets. I'll see you on the ball field.

JOHNNY MAYERS

I bowl with this next guy, JOHNNY MAYERS, and if you saw him, you would immediately know he stays in shape and is very active. Go, Johnny.

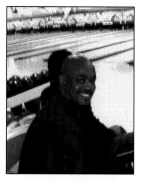

Johnny Mayers

I am Johnny R. Mayers Sr., and am 6'2" and weigh approximately 235 lbs.

Tony, you're right, I am a very active person. I am 45 years of age and have been active all my life, and have maintained my weight for many years. I see you at bowling every week and that's probably the least active sport that I'm involved in.

Actually my full-time job keeps me in shape, as I do very heavy lifting throughout the day. Two years ago (2005) I studied to be a personal trainer and now work part time as a trainer for the Sports Authority. On Sundays in football season, I play quarterback in a two-handed touch football league, and Tuesdays and Thursday nights I am an assistant coach for twelve to thirteen-year-olds in an AAU basketball league. On Wednesday nights I bowl with my wife in a co-ed bowling league. I also play basketball in an over-35 league in basketball season. In between most of this, I train very extensively at the gym with weights. My diet consists of beer and whatever my wife cooks for me. (She's a great cook.)

I am the proud father of three children and am proud of the fact that my record (number three on the all-time scoring list in basketball) for Jersey City State College still stands.

95

Wow, John, you certainly are active, and you had to have scored an awful lot of points for that record to stand for so many years. Keep it up. I'll see you at the bowling alley.

TOMMY MICHAELS

TOMMY MICHAELS has been playing ball with me for many years, as well as assisting managing. His ideas for fitness are unique and work for many people. He is still playing baseball and softball so he must be doing something right. Let's hear "The Tommy Michaels Story."

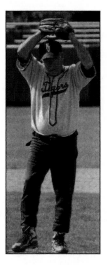

Tommy Michaels

I have enjoyed almost perfect health all my life up until age 68. Then I had a four-part bypass operation – the first time I was ever in a hospital in my entire life! In less than four months after the surgery, I was sliding into second base and back on my schedule of over 150 games a season.

My story is quite simple. But, before I begin, let me tell you about my first love: baseball.

I have always loved baseball, from that first game in late 1946 to the present. When I went with the New Jersey team to Pittsburgh in 2005, it was my 60th straight year of playing baseball and/or softball... wow! Incidentally, our team won the Bronze Medal in Over 70 Division Softball. I was unable to play the series because of a hip problem that limited me to only play 50 to 60 games during the whole season, but I coached and helped the manager, Bernie Salinger, and the team bring home the Bronze Medal.

Unlike most of my fellow baseball and softball players here in Northern New Jersey, I did not grow up in a city such as New York or Newark, but rather a small town that back in 1934 was one of many rural New Jersey towns that had more cows than people. All my brothers and sisters and I were born at home.

Luckily I had two older brothers who had me in the back yard since I was six years old, throwing baseballs while one played catcher and the other stood at the "plate" (which was the weekly newspaper folded to the size of a plate with a rock on it). From there they would hit me grounders, fly balls, and their version of batting practice. When I got to be thirteen years old, I had my first ever baseball uniform and played on a team with my brothers where the average age was nineteen! (Incidentally, I still wear that old-fashioned, heavy-cotton, button-down-the-front uniform top at least once at every baseball tournament I have played in over the past sixty-plus years. I even got some newspaper write-ups when appearing in that old 1946 Boston Braves look-alike uniform top.)

I have been playing every year since those first Saturday and Sunday doubleheaders throughout the late 1940s and into the early 1950s throughout New Jersey, Pennsylvania, and New York. It was quite a thrill for me as a young kid playing shortstop on a team of all older guys and going to all these "distant" ball fields and playing before some pretty good crowds, especially on Sundays. Then after the games, both teams would go to the local gin-mill where the home team hung out, and there would be a buffet with all kinds of food, etc. Of course, my two brothers made sure I wasn't served any harder drink than ginger ale!

I played exclusively baseball until I was 41. It got to be too competitive, as I was playing with guys literally twenty years my junior. My two oldest sons were nineteen and twenty at the time and played softball on both a local town team and a traveling team, and they invited me to join them. I did and for about ten years I played with them. Then my kids said they were 'too old' to play anymore (hey, what about me?), so I joined an over-fifty league (two nights a week); a Tuesday retirement league team (doubleheaders);

an over-sixty Saturday league team (doubleheaders); a baseball team that practices and sometimes plays on Thursdays; and an over-sixty night league team as well. In the past twenty years I have always played between a low of 40 to 50 games and a high of 160 games a year!

Now I would like to share with you how all this happened and how this information will hopefully help you and your loved ones lead a more active and healthier life! Here goes.

First off, unlike most of my ballplayer friends, I do NOT participate in too much physical exercise. What I DO and have done all my adult life is to practice PREVENTATIVE measures for my health! I have taken vitamins and minerals and other supplements since I was twenty years old! The results have been fabulous!

In addition to preventative measures, I also enjoy a very clear and upbeat mind. I rarely drink alcohol, I never smoked (my brothers would have killed me – and they smoked!), I never took any form of so-called 'recreational' or other quasi-legal or illegal drugs (I didn't even take an aspirin until I was 68!). Hence I have not polluted my mind or my body.

Here is what I would advise persons who wish for longevity, good health, and an active lifestyle throughout their lives!

1. DO some sort of exercise. Read in this book what some of the exercises are that other athletes, as well as doctors and even a nutritionist that Tony has interviewed, are doing. (Incidentally, every player mentioned in this book is a much better ball player than I was or will ever be!)

2. DO NOT hurt your body NOR YOUR MIND by ingesting things legal and/or illegal that will break down your mind and/or your body (i.e., read the fine print on ALL your prescriptions about side effects, etc.).

3. DO take vitamins, minerals, enzymes, and other supplements that build UP your body, your immune

system, etc. to PREVENT ravages of disease upon your body and mind (i.e., don't just wait for symptoms to appear and then start to treat them! And if, unfortunately, you develop symptoms, treat the CAUSE...not the symptom!).

4. DO go and play whatever is your "baseball" or "softball" or any physical activity that you enjoy. I love playing, now at 74 years old, the same as I did when I was in the backyard with my brothers almost 70 years ago!

And please let me add this. After playing ball continuously in SEVEN DECADES, I have NEVER been an outstanding player. I was constantly a good fielder but constantly a lousy hitter who always batted 9th – even back in the 'old days.' But what I have lacked in talent, I have made up with enthusiasm, hustle, knowing the game, loving the game, and always being a team player. Anyone can do this.

I hope this article helps you so you can help others too.

Tom, you certainly have given us good information, and you failed to say you have great managerial skills. While you assisted me managing over the years, we won many games and I certainly appreciated your many skills, and you underestimate your ability. I've seen you get many key hits and have even won a few games for us. You can play on my team anytime.

STEVEN NATURALE

I also interviewed my son, STEVEN NATURALE. He is somewhat of a fitness nut like me. I guess the apple doesn't fall far from the tree. Let's hear it, Steve.

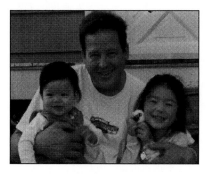

Steven Naturale

I am 5'10" and weigh approximately 185 pounds. I attribute staying in good shape to a variety of things. Working in the garment center in NYC forces me to walk quite a bit five days a week. I also work out four days a week consisting of 30 to 40 minutes of cardio (stationary bike and jog on the treadmill) and twenty minutes of circuit weight training on my chest, arms, back, triceps, and lats. I also play in an over-35 lacrosse league one night per week. But probably for me the most difficult part of staying in shape is eating correctly. I try to eat four to five small meals per day, but occasionally slack off. I look at it like this: you can always do better at eating correctly. When I eat right I feel much better, and I know what the good foods are but sometimes it's tough to stay away from the not-so-good ones, and I know I have to change my eating habits.

To sum it up, I played college football and lacrosse (graduated 1981) at 185, today I fluctuate between 190 and 195. Okay, Dad, get going on your book, maybe it will help me to eat better.

Hey Steve, maybe you should listen to your dad more. But I know you will be fifty years old soon and when you get to be my age, you will probably write your own book on fitness. And don't forget the strength and fitness program you and your cousin, Rich Tobin, are running for Montclair High School. Teaching and guiding these youngsters with a rigorous training program should keep you guys in great shape.

PAUL OLIVER

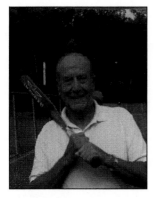

Paul Oliver

PAUL OLIVER is another ball player whom I interviewed. Paul is 81 years of experience and is still playing ball twice a week, and also plays on a tournament team that travels around the U.S.A. He grew up in St. Louis, next door to Yogi Berra. Looks like that street in St. Louis produced great athletes – Joe Garagiola from the St. Louis Cardinals baseball team also lived on that street.

Paul Oliver also played in the minor leagues with Stan Musial and other baseball greats. He has 13 championship tournament rings and was voted into the "Softball Hall of Fame." His overall tournament batting average is an amazing .863.

Paul tries to do 50 push-ups every day and does other calisthenics and stretching to stay in shape. He carefully watches his diet, and his weight has been the same for many years. If you saw him, you would never think he was 80 (81 now). He is a very active person and will play in the Senior Olympics in Kentucky for the 75-and-over team in 2007.

[Note: Paul did play in the Senior Olympics in 2007 and his team, captained by this author, won the Gold Medal for the State of New Jersey. Paul and Rich Palmer played an integral part in us winning all four games. They both batted an amazing .823. Congratulations to all of the New Jersey Embers. Now let's get ready for the next Senior Olympics in San Francisco in 2009.]

RICH PALMER

The next guy is another ballplayer that I have played with for many years. He not only has played, he is one of the players who started the seniors league. This is what RICH PALMER had to say about fitness.

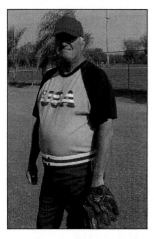

Rich Palmer

I am Rich Palmer, age 78, and I believe fitness is an obligation you make to yourself, to set up a regimen that will keep you in shape, as long as possible. Part of fitness is your keeping those fellow ball players, especially the ones in charge, knowing what obligations you will live by. Make every effort to always keep others apprised of your activity, and attendance on a timely constant basis. These same efforts will keep you in shape, as you establish exercise habits that keep you in top condition. By meeting the schedules you commit to, you will be taking care of your health.

Sometimes, at peak ball playing time, early mornings are required for you to get yourself in gear to be ready for participation. If you have trained yourself to initiate an exercise regimen prior to each game or practice, that will help you maintain the best physical condition that your age and body can handle. Obviously, the more active you are and the more competition you enter into, the more constant good health you will attain. One advantage of living in Florida is the year-round weather, which allows you to play ball or any sport throughout the twelve months. Sometimes, as we get older, it is hard to crank up the old body, but sticking to your schedule keeps you on target. You are only as old as you feel, or something like that. Health issues sometimes slow you down, but if your "fitness" schedule has been strong and constant, that may go a long way in minimizing unexpected health problems.

Finally, setting a good example in the overall "fitness" efforts will help inspire your fellow ball players, thereby making your team and group a stronger contingent. Personally, for me to stay fit is to stick with whatever I sign up for. Neither wind nor rain nor storm will stave the die-hard softball player from that which he has committed to. The hardest part is to get out of bed at 6 a.m. to be on the ball field by 8 a.m. At my age, getting in motion is sometimes hard to do. You cannot make excuses, you just have to get UP and get GOING. Once you start cutting corners, you begin to find ways to have other priorities. Do not let your body atrophy: keep it in shape and remember, "You are what you eat."

Well, I agree. Rich, you are a die-hard ball player and a darn good one. You not only can pitch, you can hit too, and you certainly have set the example for younger players. It has been a pleasure playing with you in the Senior Olympics, and I hope you can pitch and hit for our team in San Francisco in 2009.

JAY RENNIE

JAY RENNIE is a good friend of my granddaughter (Katie Hurley – see her interview) and seems to be a very focused and dedicated young man. Let's hear it from Jay.

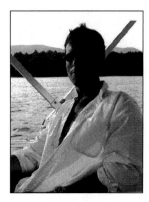

Jay Rennie

This summer I'll hit a milestone; that is, I will enter my third decade! Yet today I feel as good as, if not better than, I did in my early twenties. New acquaintances routinely think I'm five years younger than I actually am, I rarely have aches or pains despite my overly active lifestyle, and my head is always clear and focused. I place the credit for all this largely upon what I would describe as my healthy lifestyle. The essence of my routine is to keep things relatively simple. Sure, I hit the gym two to three times per week to strength train with free weights and I bike, run, swim, and canoe, but I also try to incorporate vigorous activity whenever I can. I take stairs instead of the elevator and walk whenever possible. I'm lucky enough to live within a twenty-minute walk of work, the bank, supermarket, and gym. Not only do I keep active but I'm also helping the planet by not driving as much (not to mention the cost of wear and tear on my car!).

But exercise is not everything. I make nearly all my food from scratch and try to cook and process food as little as possible: breads, pies (crust and all), hummus, curries, pasta sauces, soups, and a host of other recipes from fresh and if possible local and/or organic ingredients. Perhaps my biggest secret is taking advantage of those little invisible organisms – bacteria and yeast. These organisms (the safe ones, like safe mushrooms) produce many beneficial compounds such as essential amino acids, B-complex vitamins, intact enzymes, and also act as probiotics to keep the digestive system functioning properly. I drink Kombucha (an ancient method of fermenting tea), Kefir (cultured milk, a little like yogurt but includes yeast), use nutritional yeast (has a nutty, cheese-like flavor), eat tempeh (fermented soybeans; an excellent nutty flavor) and unfiltered and unpasteurized cider vinegar and beer. The key to these items (except nutritional yeast) is that they are unfiltered and unpasteurized, processes which can destroy many of the beneficial aspects these foods possess.

Regular exercise, fresh, minimally processed food, lots of fresh brewed tea (not the sweetened stuff you buy), plenty of liquids, and a daily 10-20 minute stretching routine has worked extremely well for me. It is not always easy to incorporate such lifestyle choices, but in my book the results translate into better sleep and more energy during the day and so better productivity overall. Even as I enter my thirties, I routinely out-compete younger peers, sleep well, have stable moods, and rarely if ever suffer aches and pains.

Thanks, Jay, I like your routine and especially like your attitude about eating and exercise. You should be around for many decades.

JOHN REYNOLDS

JOHN REYNOLDS, the son of my good friends Betty and Jimmy Nasisi, is a physician's assistant, nutritionist and herbalist, and has his own medical practice. Let's hear your story, John.

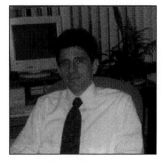

John Reynolds

I am a graduate of the Physician Assistant program at SUNY Stony Brook. I also hold a degree in Biology and Nutrition. I have been in practice for 25 years. I work for a holistic physician and in addition I own a small medical practice of my own. At age 54 I weigh 157 lbs., standing 5'8½" tall. I have a fairly muscular physique, having weight trained for nearly forty years. My body fat is approximately 15%. While not world class, I have encountered many patients who are 30%, 40% or even 50% body fat. To keep myself in this condition, I practice rigorous nutritional principles. I repeatedly, tell my patients, "I DO NOT CONTROL MY WEIGHT IN THE GYM, I CONTROL MY WEIGHT IN THE KITCHEN."

- I cook virtually all my own food seven days a week.
- I eat no refined foods (fast foods, frozen entrees).
- I strictly avoid sugars in all forms (no cookies, candies, cakes, ice cream, sodas, etc.).
- I do not smoke. I consume no alcohol. I have no caffeine.
- I do not eat gluten-containing grains (wheat, rye, barley, and oats).

- I weigh and measure my carbohydrate-containing foods, keeping my carbs to within 150 grams per day.
- I rotate my diet, meaning I do not eat the same foods every day.
- I eat a salad that would provide a good-sized serving for four people (I make it in a pasta bowl and it's completely full) every day.
- There is more, however. I think you see that I am quite committed. My folks, who have taken me to restaurants and watched me eat, can certainly verify much of what I am telling you.
- My exercise and supplement regimen are variable, depending on how I feel and what I think I need.
- Typically I will start the day with 1 Tbsp of psyllium powder in water sweetened with Stevia. This promotes normal bowel function and also helps to lower cholesterol.
- Then ½ teaspoon of acidophilus powder to enhance the normal flora in the intestine and suppress the growth of yeast.
- Vitamin D 1000 IU 2 X daily – this helps promote healthy bones and also fights various cancers.
- St. John's Wort liquid, three drops in water for mood enhancement.
- Biotin 1000 mcg, one daily for healthy hair, skin and nails.
- Horse chestnut seed extract, one cap three times weekly for healthy veins.
- Hemp oil, 1 Tbsp for skin and hair health.
- Vitamin E 400 most days for blood thinning, anti-aging.
- Digestive enzymes with most meals to promote healthy digestion and absorption.
- Various joint formulas with herbs, glucosamine and chondroitin for joint repair.
- Iodine liquid (not available OTC) to promote healthy

thyroid functioning.

- DHEA liquid (by prescription), three to five drops daily to help with adrenal function.
- Apricot kernels – I chew about eight a day for their high laetrile content – some holistic practitioners believe this helps fight off any cancer cells that may be forming in the body.
- Calcium and magnesium for healthy bones, muscles and nerves.
- Vitamin A 25,000, one cap three times weekly for skin, immune system.
- Melatonin, 2 mg, for sleep.

There are other supplements I use as needed, such as chelating agents to remove toxic metals, special B vitamin formulations, natural antihistamines for allergies, certain multivitamin preparations and others, but the above is my regular protocol.

For physical activity, I both weight train and take care of my house. Since I own my own home, I do a lot of physical labor taking care of the grounds. For example, I purposely bought a lawn mower that is not self-propelled and is a pull-start to increase my physical output. I may spend several hours doing manual labor such as mopping floors, mowing the lawn, trimming bushes, etc. Sometimes I follow this activity with a workout. I have put together a small gym in my basement. I will typically start with a rebounder (mini trampoline) on which I run in place for several minutes for a warm-up. I do a lot of dumbbell work because they allow muscle groups to go through their complete natural range of motion and do not restrict you as bars, some cables and machines do.

I do three to four sets of dumbbell side laterals for the deltoids and also three to four sets of dumbbell curls for the biceps. I may also do dumbbell rowing for the lats. This gives a nice sweep to the upper body. I also do three to four sets of lying flies for the pectorals. In between sets I will often do push-ups to keep my pulse rate up. I do a special dumbbell movement that works the "core" muscles. The dumbbell is raised up and down from the chest to overhead while simultaneously squatting (has to be demonstrated). I also do abdominal work, including incline sit-ups, decline leg raises and side bends. I also own a total gym and will alternate my workouts with that at times or combine it with barbell work. I will exercise three to six times weekly and therefore the entire body is worked out every week.

Finally and most importantly, there is my spiritual connection. In order to be well, one must seek out a relationship with the ALMIGHTY. The soul must be fed as well as the body. To do this, I pray morning and evening, read the Bible daily and attend church weekly. Anyone of any faith can incorporate these principles. My final piece of wisdom: If you have God in your heart and good food in your body, you cannot fail.

—John J. Reynolds, PA-C, CCN

Wow, John, I particularly like that statement, "I DO NOT CONTROL MY WEIGHT IN THE GYM, I CONTROL MY WEIGHT IN THE KITCHEN." How true, and of course it's not a bad idea to stay linked to the ALMIGHTY. You certainly practice what you preach. Thanks, Doctor John, see you in our "old age."

HARRY ROSENTHAL

Fellow ball player HARRY ROSENTHAL has a pretty good program going. Let's hear it, Harry.

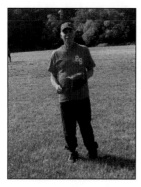

Harry Rosenthal

My mother always used to say, "Harry, age is just a number," and, even at this young age of 67 years, I would have to agree as my philosophy has become: "Keep your mind and body busy and you will continue to enjoy life to the fullest," and I've never felt better.

I wasn't always this smart but was always active. While working I played for the company softball team...when we periodically had one; a little tennis, and twenty years ago joined a gym (initially to reduce stress from marital problems), but generally only went on weekends and sometimes only one day because I was too tired at night after working in New York City each day and commuting to my home in West Orange, New Jersey. I smoked cigars but stopped that ten years ago and generally was ten to fifteen pounds overweight. I am presently 171 lbs.

As a senior who loves life, I now go to the gym at 6:00 a.m. (that's when it opens) on Monday, Wednesday and Friday and usually one day on the weekend; my habits of yesterday are a faded memory. While there I do one hour on the treadmill, various weight exercises, various arm and leg machine exercises, then go to the pool area for the pool, whirlpool, steam room or sauna. In addition, I have made many friends at the gym but I always make sure I have my complete workout. I find it amazing when I hear someone who comes to the gym to work out complaining that they had to just walk too far from their parking space.

On days that I don't go to the gym or play softball, I usually take a one-to-two-mile walk. In fact, when in New York City, where I go fairly often, I always prefer walking up to two or three miles to subways and to cabs. Each day I make sure I have some form of physical exercise, and I still shovel snow and mow my grass (fortunately I don't have to do both in the same day!). I play softball on Saturdays and Thursdays, weather permitting, throughout the year except for extreme winter conditions.

As far as vitamins, I never took any until about five years ago as a close, lifelong friend, who is a doctor, told me in order to reduce the risk of cancer and heart problems, take daily: vitamin C, vitamin E, folic acid and an aspirin, as well as glucosamine and chondroitin for joint lubrication/ arthritis. Since I began this regime I have noticed almost a complete reduction in discomfort. This doesn't have the same positive result for everyone, but, like chicken soup, it can't hurt.

As far as my eating habits, I have lost about 10 pounds and have kept most of it off. I used to eat a bagel and butter every morning and then one day, I thought of 30 of them stacked up, and I chose to eliminate them. When I see my weight going up, I immediately go on a modified South Beach Diet…basically eliminate all things white. There is a joy to my focus of sharing. See you all in our old age…

Thanks, Harry, sounds pretty good – keep it up.

DON ROTH

DON ROTH, a fellow ball player, has a very inspirational story. Let's hear it, Don. (And another guy that came from Brooklyn.)

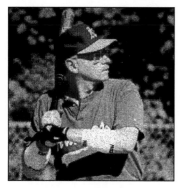

Don Roth

It was a cool morning in November 2001 as I walked the three blocks from my parking lot to my Brooklyn office. As I walked that November morning I felt a strange sensation in my chest. It disappeared at work but on my walk back that evening, the feeling returned. This persisted for three weeks when I finally decided to see a doctor. After many tests, the doctor recommended that I see a cardiologist. I said, "What!!"

Three weeks later I was in the hospital having an angiogram, which immediately led to an angioplasty and the installation of two stents to open two blocked arteries. The cardiologist informed me that I had seven blockages that he would attempt to control with diet and exercise. Needless to say, I was just given tremendous motivation to change my eating habits and exercise routines.

So, in January 2002, I began greatly reducing the saturated fat in my diet. No more hot dogs, hamburgers, pizza, cheeses, cakes, cookies, butter, dark chocolate raisins (which I love), and all other chocolate candy (how very depressing!). My daughter, a personal trainer, developed a workout regimen for me and convinced me to start using

114

my Soloflex resistance machine, which I only used to hang up my shirts, and instead use it for what it was intended.

Still working in Brooklyn and leaving my house each morning at 4:50 a.m. and returning home at 7:30 p.m. made it difficult to follow my diet and especially exercise regularly. I did the best I could and anxiously prepared for my team's first softball practice in late March. Needless to say, it was great getting out there the first day and seeing all the guys and just doing it. Unfortunately, on the ride home I felt discomfort in the left side of my chest. As soon as I arrived home and my wife saw me, she, despite my protests, immediately called 911. Two weeks later, at Morristown Memorial Hospital, I had triple bypass open heart surgery. My softball season was over but my new way of life had begun.

I retired on July 1, 2003 and never looked back. I follow my diet pretty carefully, even shying away from softball pizza and chicken wing luncheons. I now have my Soloflex machine, a treadmill and a stationary bike in my basement. My personal trainer has me doing 50 chest flies, 50 upright rows, 50 biceps curls and 50 squats at least three days a week. In addition, I'm on the treadmill for thirty minutes or, during softball season, to take pressure off my legs, 30 minutes on the stationary bike. In addition, during the summer, I do laps in my pool and kayak regularly.

At age 63, 6 feet tall and 195 pounds, I've never felt better. Since retirement, life has been just great. I realize work is a means to an end, but compared to retirement – well, there is no comparison. I love spending more time with my family and absolutely love softball. I originally played more than 75 games a year, with leagues on Saturdays, Tuesday mornings and evenings during the week, plus a fall league. I have since given up the Tuesdays to watch my grandchildren, which is simply wonderful.

So, from being a 57-year-old guy who almost suddenly dropped dead from a fatal heart attack, I have gone on to be a 63-year-old who is in pretty good shape, who exercises regularly, eats well and is totally enjoying life. In my softball career I am inspired by men such as the author of this book and his buddies, who are still playing competitively into their seventies and eighties. I should be so lucky!!

Don't wait to feel that uncomfortable feeling in your chest. Exercise and eat well now. Enjoy!!!!

Wow, Don, that's a great inspirational story, and I hope that many people will take heed of it and follow your advice to get in shape, eat right and not wait until it's too late. I know we will see you on the ball field for many years to come. Keep it up.

JERRY RUSSO

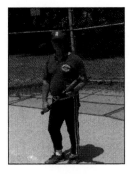

Jerry Russo

JERRY RUSSO, another ball player, at age 72 is in great shape. He was a soccer player and is actually a member of the New Jersey Soccer Hall of Fame. Although Jerry says he doesn't have a regular regimen of exercises, he is very active. In high school he played soccer, basketball and baseball, and started playing softball at a very young age – he sometimes plays six softball games a week. And the only time he gained a great amount of weight was when he had a knee replacement a few years ago. Many days he will play two games during the day and then another one at night.

After his knee replacement he seemed to run faster than he originally did; in fact, he's the reason I had my replacement. I didn't want to do it, assuming I wouldn't be able to continue playing, but like Jerry, I think I run faster than before the operation.

Jerry says he eats very few desserts and watches his diet very carefully, and doesn't have time to gain weight. While a teacher, he coached soccer and actually scrimmaged with the players.

Two years ago Jerry played in the over-seventy-year-old Senior Olympics in Pittsburgh and was voted "The Most Valuable Player," and his New Jersey seventies team, coached by Bernie Salinger, won the Bronze Medal. Okay, Jerry, keep it up and I know I'll see you on the ball fields for many more years.

CLIF SEIPAL

A good friend of mine and fellow Montclair High Schooler CLIF SEIPAL has an unorthodox way of staying fit. (You do whatever works for you.) He is an engineer and a pretty bright guy, so I think we should listen to what he has to say. Go, Clif.

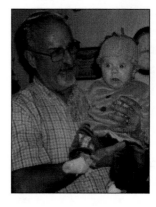
Clif Seipal

Brain exercises: Daily including weekends – Sudoku, "Word-Roundup" and jigsaw puzzles as presented on www.AARPmagazine.org/games, as well as daily paper's Sudoku.

Exercise: YES – BUT NO WEIGHTS or GYMS!!!!!! I cut the grass, split wood, rake leaves, shovel snow, build rock walls: EXERCISE with **byproduct OUTPUT!!** More inclined toward endurance vs. POWER!!!

As a kid, I grew up at Lake Mohawk lakefront during summers when not cutting our and neighbors' lawns or cutting down trees, removing stumps, refilling holes with dirt and reseeding for $15 per tree. No power saw – only manual tools!! And boating – we had a kayak (homemade), canoe, rowboat and sailboat. BUT NO MOTORS – instead paddles, oars, sails!!!!! And while we were at the lake, we would swim laps in our 1000-foot-wide cove and also swim across the lake to beach on opposite shore (5/8 mile) while a brother paddled the canoe alongside. The roles were reversed for the return trip. I still own Sunfish and Lightning sailboats! A 100-year-old twin oak came down due to a hurricane. Dad could have bought a chainsaw – BUT – NO!!!! Having three sons and subscribing to "a kid who is busy hasn't time to get into trouble," Mom enforced his instruction that each son spend four hours a day with his brothers at the ends of a six-foot two-man SAW. I still have the SAW!!!!! Seven days a week reduced the tree, branches and all, to a couple cords of wood which then had to be split. It took several weeks, and what a pile of wood for the fireplace it was. I still maintain my yards and veggie gardens (reminds me – got to get a new Rototiller carburetor for a couple years!!!). I have adopted a dog and go on daily walks of two to four miles, weather permitting. Corki's litter patrols again have **BYPRODUCT value** as I can't stand litter on neighborhood streets. I have twelve different Montville routes and two at the shore to vary the scenery and coverage.

Coaching soccer: (twenty plus years) Kept away from the "beer locker" two nights a week. I also wouldn't ask the team to do any exercise/skill that I wouldn't do with them.

Fitness: At the shore, I would go surf casting. Among the wave action up to the waist strengthened the muscles about the spine while enjoying the activity. Never caught any fish, as would only have a lead weight attached – no hooks or bait. It was great for unconsciously strengthening the spine.

Rx/Meds: NONE! Not even vitamins.

Alcohol: Daily BEERS – infrequently wines – whiskey sours at annual ITT Quarter Century Dinner/Dance and weddings. I also have beer when working on hot days. It has great hydration value.

WEIGHT (obesity): In 1973, months after our first daughter's birth, I suffered a herniated disk. When the weight gets beyond 200 lbs. (holiday time is tough), exacerbations occur, but the fast daily dog walks over irregular terrain seem to have given me a 10 to 12 lb. buffer.

And **FOOD:** I love fresh veggies – broccoli, bell peppers, carrots, cauliflower, cucumbers, beans with dip!!! I also prefer to snack on fresh fruit or nuts – DID TONY SAY I WAS

NUTS????? Must be you are what you eat

We grew up with NATURAL FOODS – much home-grown and homemade!!!! Very little candy and junk food. The "fastest food" was in the country with hot dogs and hamburgers made over a fire using dead branches collected from the lawn. No charcoal or propane, as we were recovering from the Depression. You had to finish your plate OR NO DESSERT!!!!! To this day I'd rather have a second helping and forego the desserts. That's my story...

Clif, no meds at your age – that's great. That's one thing you and I have in common, and your exercise regimen is as good as any weightlifter's and maybe better. I would recommend some vitamins, but if it's not broken, no need to worry. You are a man in motion – keep it up. (And you're not nuts – me either.)

TOM SHANNON

In spite of predicted inclement weather, yesterday was cause for celebration as my manuscript was finished. My wife, Madeline; my editor, Grange, and I happily had put my manuscript together to drop off to Patty Shannon, owner (along with husband Brian) of The Wordstation, a unique secretarial business located in Avon-by-the-Sea, New Jersey, to authors from all over the United States. I might add, the Shannons are also Montclair State alumni, my alma mater. Patty had typed and set up my last book for publishing and I was very pleased with everything she did.

While having a seafood lunch down by the water, Grange, having known Patty for over fifteen years, told us about Patty and Brian's son, TOM SHANNON, a truly amazing handsome, fit and athletic autistic child. Knowing he is a little different than his peers, but unconcerned about it, he goes about his life with a joi de vivre we could all aspire to. I listened and realized Tom's young life is so inspirational that I felt my readers should hear it. Not only is he "fit" at the ever young age of eighteen, he is an amazing person. Let's hear the story, Patty:

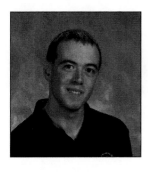

Tom Shannon

My son, Tom, was diagnosed with autism in 1993, about three months before his third birthday. At that time it was not as common for a pediatrician to recognize the signs of autism as early as mine did, and I will be forever grateful to him for pushing to have Tom tested. After we got over the first devastation and grief of the diagnosis, we were determined to put everything we had into helping Tom go as far in this life as he could. I gave up my idea of going back to work when he started school, and began a home business as a professional proofreader and word processor. Over the next few years, this turned out to be successful enough to move the business out of our home and into a retail space in town, and eventually allowed my husband, Brian, to quit corporate life and join me in the business, which he expanded into offering cards and gifts as well as the original secretarial services. Although owning a business can be risky financially, being able to set our own schedules and make sure we were there for Tom when he needed us, and to get him to therapies and other activities, was worth more than any amount of money.

We wanted Tom to be physically fit as well, but discovered early on that team sports were NOT the way to go. The noise and confusion, the competitiveness, the rushed pace were all overwhelming to a child with autism. Since I had taken tap lessons on and off through most of my life, I hesitantly approached the local dance studio and asked if they would give Tom a chance. He started out taking private lessons but very soon was included in the regular classes. He turned out to have an excellent memory and a great sense of rhythm. Because one of the hallmarks of autism is a lack of social awareness, he had no issues with being one of only two boys in the dance school. The girls thought it was fun to have a boy in their class. For many years he took jazz, tap and ballet lessons. He only gave it up when he started high school and his schedule there made it difficult to fit in the dance classes, although he still takes lessons every summer. And to this day the girls in his old classes will run over to say hello to Tom when they see him.

We also found that Special Olympics gymnastics classes were a wonderful outlet, and one of the local gymnastics places was an active participant. He spent three or four years with them, and has the medals to show for it! One year we were even fortunate enough to be sponsored by the local PBA.

Tom was unable to ride a bicycle for a long time, both because of coordination problems and because it would not be safe for him, since he couldn't split his attention enough to watch for traffic. So Brian bought a tandem bike, and for many years he and Tom could be seen all up and down the shore riding together. My contribution was to take him bowling, roller skating and ice skating. Anything to keep him off the couch, or away from the computer! I had seen too many developmentally disabled children becoming obese because of lack of exercise. (Luckily, Tom never required any kind of medications that can cause weight gain.) Tom also, as he matured and became more aware of his surroundings, was able to walk more on his own, and even safely ride a bicycle. Also, Brian took over cooking duties several years ago, and provides healthy meals to keep us all on track.

We have been blessed with wonderful teachers and therapists over the years, and Tom is now a happy, healthy eighteen-year-old, finishing up his junior year in the local high school, where he is fully mainstreamed and is an honor student. He participates in chorus and in drama club. He is a kind, caring young man and his classmates have accepted him without reservations. I'd like to end with a paragraph from an essay Tom wrote about himself for his English class:

"We all know that we are unique in every way and have some type of talent. Here are some things that are unique about me. I have a developmental disability called Autism. That means my brain works differently, and I have trouble socializing and speaking. But in some ways, I'm able to develop many different skills and do a lot of things without worrying about this disability. For example, I took dance classes for many years. Despite the fact that I was the only boy in my classes and one of only two boys in the whole school, I specialized in ballet, jazz, and tap dancing. I also have a love of music and have somehow developed perfect pitch, which not a lot of people have, including other musicians. One of my other interests is in foreign languages, which is partly why I take Spanish and French courses at school and own many different phrasebooks on foreign languages. I also like to travel to different places. Those are the things that make me special, and I am happy to say that I am doing very well in life so far thanks to my wonderful family in the neighborhood in New Jersey that I love, the great education I received from different schools, and the wonderful friends I have that have helped me in getting through the courses of my life. What a wonderful world I'm living in! Let's keep it that way!"

Wow, Patty, what an amazing story. Both you and Brian are to be highly commended for your love, devotion, perseverance and dedication, defying the odds as you stayed focused and dared to, with the aid of family and friends, be a "typical" family. I am truly honored to have the Shannon family as part of my book... God bless you all.

BILL SMITH

I interviewed "BILL SMITH" today, January 12, 2005 (some names are fictitious). Bill is 79 years of age and is an actuary. He's not in very good shape and he knows it. He's about 5'11" and weighs about 230 lbs. No, he's not a wrestler – well, yes he is, in a way – he wrestles with numbers, but he has been retired a few years and really doesn't do too much exercise. He says in the summer time he does a lot of gardening work, which is the extent of his exercise.

One good thing is he used to smoke for many years and has given that up. He says he feels much better since he stopped smoking. So why is he in the fitness book? I stated earlier I am going to use anyone who can help us to get on a program. You see, Bill has finally realized he has to do something or he won't last too long. He's an intelligent man and I bet when he reads this whole book, he will try even harder to get in shape. Bill believes most of staying fit comes from genetics, but is now trying to diet also. I explained to him that he must do diet and exercise, and yes, your genes do play a part in your overall fitness. But I will tell you right now, I don't care how good your genes are: if you are not dieting and exercising enough, you will not be fit. That's not just coming from me, that's from almost every health book I have perused.

Bill stated when he was going to NYC to his job every day, he was doing a lot of walking, and was probably doing enough of it to keep him in fairly good shape. Since he's retired, he's gained a lot of weight. Bill is like many very unfit people who retire and their lifestyle changes. He now has eliminated white bread and sugar and sweets from his diet and is attempting to bring his weight down.

I had stated earlier that we would use the process of elimination in an attempt to assist the reader to get into some type of program to improve their fitness. Well, we can learn from Bill Smith. What is he doing right and what is he doing wrong? We try and retain the good stuff and eliminate the bad. He has eliminated the smoking – that's good. He's not doing much exercise at all in the winter – that, of course, is bad. I would like to see him just start slowly with maybe 15 minutes a day of stretching and light calisthenics, then work up to one hour a day. He should continue his walking every day, even if it's only ten minutes to start, but eventually work it up gradually as his weight goes down, which it will because he has also cut down on his diet. He states he has vegetable portions every day – now that's good. I would like to see him supplement between-meals fruit, on a daily basis, and before every meal drink a large glass of water or skim milk. This will curb his appetite and he won't eat as much as usual… Of course, as I've stated earlier, write everything down daily, so you can actually see what you did the previous day.

Okay, Bill, I know this book won't be done in two months so I'll check with you then and see how you're doing... Good luck.

Note: I checked with Bill three months after the interview and he had lost 10 lbs. and was doing some type of exercise every other day. He said he feels much better and will continue to diet and exercise.

ROGER SPAIN

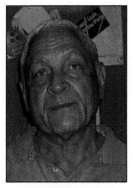

Roger Spain

I also interviewed ROGER SPAIN. Roger worked with me as a police officer and has been retired for quite a few years now. He is 69 years old and is in excellent condition. If you saw him you would immediately know he lifts weights and stays in great shape. He states he works out three days a week with heavy weights doing curls, bicep exercises and bench presses. His workout lasts 1½ hours every Tuesday, Thursday and Saturday. Roger also is active in bowling and other physical activities and keeps a strict diet. He is a solid 205 lbs. for his 5'11" frame. Roger was an excellent softball player while on the police department and I'm working on him to play in our "seniors" league for the Senior Olympics. Good luck, Roger. Keep up the good work and I hope to see you on the ball field.

GENE STRACCO

GENE STRACCO, a fellow ball player, has been playing and coaching for many years. Let's hear what he has to say...

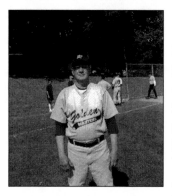

Gene Stracco

I have been involved with sports for almost my entire life. I remember my father putting on my first baseball glove when I was three, and my passion for competitive sports has never waned. As I was growing up, I followed all the baseball teams in New York – the Yankees, Giants, and Dodgers. After the World Series was over, I rooted for the football Giants, and during the winter, the Knicks. In high school I played basketball and baseball, and in college I participated in intramural sports. I chose teaching as my career and eventually coached baseball and basketball. I took pride in my conditioning and the conditioning of my ball players. We lifted weights, ran sprints, took long runs prior to the season, watched the diets, etc. All the good things coaches do for themselves and their players to keep in good shape

At the beginning of the 1978 basketball season at Randolph High School, I was demonstrating how to pivot left and drive to the basket when suddenly, I felt a snap, like a thin piece of wood breaking in half. It was my Achilles tendon!!! I was in excruciating pain. I tried to get up but could not support my weight. The orthopedic surgeon said I had completely ruptured the tendon and it had to be surgically repaired. He described it as a broken rubber band with dangling ends. I coached that entire season with my left leg in a cast.

In 1991, I was a high school administrator in the Roxbury Township school system. In March of that year, the student council arranged a volleyball tournament to benefit a particular charity. All components of the school system had representative teams: the board of education, high school administrators, the teachers, each elementary school, and the students. While I was playing, I tried to spike the ball, and in mid-air, I felt the same "snap." This time it was my right leg and, again, the Achilles was completely ruptured. After the surgery and rehab, the surgeon said the only form of exercise I should follow is walking. How boring!!!

I have been playing softball for thirty years. The last seventeen years I have been playing with two surgically repaired Achilles tendons. At 64, I am still running, batting, diving for balls, and loving it. To keep in shape, I go to the gym every other day when I am not playing ball, stretch the Achilles every day, lift weights, and watch my diet. I have fresh fruit and vegetables every day, no red meat, eliminated caffeine. During the winter, I still go the gym, jog about two miles on the treadmill, stretch and stretch, and go to Florida to play ball. My wife thinks I am crazy, but when you have softball "fever" nothing stops you, not even repaired legs.

Boy, Gene, many people would have given up after such serious injuries, but your perseverance has paid off and here you are, still playing a "boy's" game. Your exercise routine has paid off for you and I am honored to be playing ball with you.

BOB THOUROT

I've been playing ball with BOB THOUROT for over five years now and since he had a hip replacement, he has become quite a physical specimen and one of the better ball players in our seniors league. But let's let him tell you. Go, Bob.

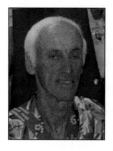

Bob Thourot

Since my hip injury about five years ago, I have tried to stay healthy by exercising daily. When home in NJ, usually from mid April to December, I try to do a lot of stretching, sit-ups and range of motion exercise (with five-pound weights) almost daily. I will do leg exercises every other day. At least two times a week I will do strength exercise for my upper body using thirty-pound weights. Also during the time period of June to September, I will swim almost every day for at least twenty minutes. I ride a bike for approximately two miles and if the weather is bad, I will use the stationary bike. During the season I will play softball three to four times a week.

When I'm in Florida from January to mid April, I do a little more swimming and bike riding. With the better weather and more time on my hands, I usually will cycle daily (with my wife) two miles in the morning and then again in the afternoon. I also do my daily stretching and exercises. While in Florida I will play two nine-inning softball games a week and roughly twelve tournament games over the three months. Of course I do many other physical activities, like mowing the lawn and other odd jobs.

I would like to add my wife does a tremendous job cooking healthy and wholesome foods that help to keep me in shape. My weight, 165, is what I weighed my junior year in high school, and I hope to play ball and be fit for many more years.

Bob, I know you will be playing for many more years. I sure wish I could throw the ball the way you do. And let's not forget how many athletes you have inspired and helped during your career as a physical education teacher.

DIANE VON GAL-TOBIN

I interviewed my niece, DIANE von GAL-TOBIN, a certified physical trainer in her forties who has four children – Wyatt, age 1; Nolan, 2; Vreeland, 5; and Michael, her stepson – whoops, now she has five. Ruby was just born a few minutes ago as I write. (I'm not kidding.) You can understand how busy her day is without a fitness program, so let's ask her how she does it. Go, Diane.

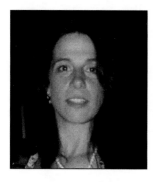

Diane Von Gal-Tobin

I am Diane von Gal-Tobin and am a 46-year-old, ever-young, proud-to-be-Mom of four fantastic kids – actually five, if you count my amazing athletically superior stepson, Michael, known as the "Pele" of lacrosse, doing hat tricks and scoring goals at most games, breaking all Montclair High School records under the astute tutelage of my darling husband, Rich, who is his coach. "Fitness" is the middle name of my entire family and eating healthy has top priority.

With those statistics stated, let me tell you a bit about what life was like before children. I always knew, from the time I was fifteen and started lifting weights and becoming quite muscular (but that was covered by a lot of fat), I wanted to compete in female body building, not as it is today but a more tender, softer version; I think it is comparable to women's fitness competitions of today. I may have been lifting, but I never changed my eating habits nor did I do any cardiovascular exercise. Although cardio is important, and I love it as it is like an injection of endorphins which allow a natural high, I early on found that eating is one of the most important factors in changing your body composition.

In my early twenties, living in New York City, I became a part of the "singles" scene in the city that never sleeps and somewhat abandoned my focus, enjoying the exposure to all types of ethnic foods and beverages. I fell in love with a young man of the same mind set and we opened up two bars in Manhattan, living an insane life that, like a fuse, short-circuited all too soon; those late nights that turned into early mornings really didn't constitute a healthy lifestyle or a healthy marriage. In spite of myself, something had to give; we parted and I went back to what was familiar...working out and running at least five miles a day. Never looking back, I joined a gym and went every day and felt that wonderful effervescent focus of getting into a zone where I wanted to be the best I could be. I had an aerobics class every morning, became a vegetarian and got a job at the gym, as I never do anything halfway.

As I began to teach people the proper way to exercise and eat, I learned a lot about myself, dropping three dress sizes; worked on mind, body and spirit, found a new apartment and, in the process, met a young man who thought he was an exercise kahoona and also thought that I just was not fit enough and not thin enough. In the process of getting to know this exercise nut case, I became an exercise "bulimic" (meaning that whenever I overate, I would do an insane amount of exercise to negate the calories I took in). I took a quantum leap into a world I knew was not right for me. I had to validate myself for me, so I "evaporated," said goodbye, never looking back, and switched jobs, going to the extreme of gaining 30 pounds. Unhappy, unfit and totally ready to focus and begin a new life, I met and fell in love with the longest drink of water (all 6'7" inches of him) who saw a woman that he thought was, as the putty cat says, "purrrrrfect."

And here I am, happily married for seven years with four

great kids, plus my fantastic fifteen-year-old bonus son, so what do I do now? Right now I joined the YMCA because they offered babysitting. Started taking cycling classes, and within a month started teaching there. I chase my children most days and am obligated to work out three days a week to teach my classes. Having this commitment is the only way I work out on a regular basis. If it weren't in my schedule, I wouldn't do it. Many a morning I would rather stay home and play with my kids, but the others need me as much as I need them.

Next month I plan to put my weightlifting program back into my regimen – one thing at a time.

Thanks, Di, keep it up and you'll keep it off. You failed to mention that you teach an intensive spin class at the YMCA.

RICHARD TOBIN

My nephew, RICHARD TOBIN, at 6'7" and 230 pounds is an imposing figure. At age 47 he's in great shape, so let's hear how he does it.

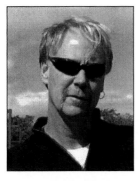

Richard Tobin

Wait a minute, Uncle Tony. Before I even get into my fitness concepts, let me tell you about my amazing, beautiful and fit wife: Diane! She is the reason I get up every day and wear a smile. Her superior genetics seem to be in glide before her feet even hit the floor – her joy of life, just attending to five kids, cleaning the house, washing the clothes, buying the right foods, cooking for our brood, keeping three dogs and two cats fed, and exercising...all while wearing a smile, mind you, would be enough for the normal person. Not so; as she is also a qualified fitness trainer who I call "Wonder Woman."

Working out started out as a way to get an athletic advantage playing high school sports. It has since evolved into a lifestyle for me. I now work out three to four times a week. I generally start with 40 minutes of cardio followed by weight training. I favor periodization and change my routine every two to three weeks. I also change the weights from heavy to low with more reps. I have found out that when I stay on track with my program, my life runs smoother and I'm definitely more focused. I cannot imagine my life without my exercise regimen. My wife, Diane (preceding interview), is a physical trainer, so we both like the same things, and she is an excellent cook so we eat very healthy foods. I say set your target and go forth for a "healthy you."

Thanks, Rich, but you failed to mention that you coach a lacrosse team, and you and Di have five children; that alone keeps you guys in motion. Also I know you and my son Steven have a fitness program going for Montclair High School students which also keeps you guys in shape.

LUKE WALSH

LUKE WALSH, a fellow bowler whom I have known for many years, is very fit for his 82 years on this planet. Let's hear Luke's story.

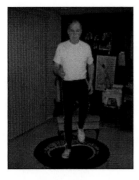
Luke Walsh

Tony, I am flattered that you have included me in your fitness book, and like you, I am also a "fitness nut."

At age 82, 5'11" and 180 lbs., I feel great and am in excellent condition. Bowling is probably the least active sport that I do.

I come from a family of twelve children. My dad was in the USN during World War I and, like you, Tony; he was a member of the Montclair Police Department for over thirty years.

Here is my routine: I set my alarm for 7 a.m. almost every morning as soon as I arise, I get on the floor and do various arm, leg and back stretches. I then stand up and do many exercises for my legs, arms and shoulders. I then go down to my family room, where I have weights, a trampoline and an ab slider. The weights range from 5 to 15 pounds and I work each exercise 10 to 15 reps. I work out 15 to 20 minutes on my trampoline and sometimes longer. Before I have breakfast I will have two glasses of water. I will then have a hearty breakfast, usually consisting of cereal, apricots, bananas, dried fruit, blueberries and grape juice. I will have a light lunch and a reasonably good dinner.

I consume approximately 21 vitamins daily and I am very active as I play golf, tennis and bowl. I am also very active with my grandchildren and travel with them a lot as they are involved in field hockey, volleyball, and roller hockey, going all over the state to various tournaments. I am a widower but enjoy a good social life as I love dancing and life in general.

I thank God for His good graces and blessings. I know my Catholic faith has a lot to do with my good health and I thank Him every morning, evening and in between.

Luke, its people like you who give us incentive to stay fit. I'm sure the readers of this book will pick that up as I certainly have. God bless you and keep dancing.

DR. ALAN WILLIAMS

Doctor ALAN WILLIAMS, a fellow Montclair High School graduate, is a cross-country bicyclist. As a doctor, he knows what you need to do to stay fit, and he certainly has applied it to his lifestyle, so let's hear from the doctor and his regimen.

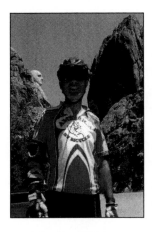

Dr. Alan Williams

I was born in New York City in 1937. My family moved from New York to Montclair in 1943 and I was a product of the Montclair public school system, spending Grades 1-9 at Mt. Hebron Elementary and Junior High School and Grades 10-12 at Montclair High. I enjoyed athletics, especially baseball, from an early age, and was a member of the baseball and basketball teams at MHS. Colgate University freshman baseball proved to all that I was "good field, no hit," and I switched to lacrosse.

Upon graduation from Colgate, I attended Navy OCS and then served on a Pacific Fleet aircraft carrier (Hancock) as a gunnery officer. It was while my ship was home-ported in the San Francisco Bay Area that I became interested in tennis, as a number of the other junior officers played tennis. I had played quite a bit of golf during high school and college years, but essentially gave up golf for tennis and am only now endeavoring to get back into golf. While in the Navy I began to run as a way to improve and maintain conditioning. Also being a member of the ship's basketball team that traveled to tournaments in Japan and the Philippines helped with conditioning.

After the Navy I spent a brief time working for a bank on Wall Street. However, during that period I became interested in the field of medicine, to the point where I made the commitment to attend medical school. I was accepted at the SUNY (formerly Syracuse University) College of Medicine in Syracuse. It was while living in upstate New York with its snowy winters that I became enamored with downhill skiing. My family and I took ski trips annually with our children and I continue to ski each winter in Colorado, Utah or British Columbia.

After my training in diagnostic radiology and neuroradiology, my family and I moved to Milwaukee, and it was in Wisconsin that I really got into road racing, mostly 5K and 10K runs but also three marathons. I would run most days, even through the heart of the Wisconsin winters. It was also in Wisconsin that I got interested in road biking. I worked up to riding a couple of centuries, as well as lesser rides. It became apparent that biking was easier on the knees and feet than running and that I should spend more time biking and less time running. A move to St. Louis underlined the idea of more biking and less running, as the summers in St. Louis were very hot and humid, which made running less enjoyable.

With all the lower body exercise that biking and running was producing, it made me feel that I was ignoring the upper body to its detriment. So, I installed a weight machine similar to a Nautilus in my basement toward the end of our stay in Wisconsin and have used it regularly (2-3 times per week) since then. I played slow-pitch softball in Milwaukee for a number of years. It was great fun but the post-game gatherings in a local tavern did not do much for participants' conditioning.

The idea of riding my bike across the U.S. began to percolate in my brain some years ago. I thought it would be a neat thing to do, but I could not get any of my riding friends to consider joining me. Working full-time was not

140

conducive to the training and participating in such a ride. But when I went from full-time to part-time at Washington University and relocated from St. Louis to NW Washington State (Blaine), the idea of a cross-country ride resurfaced. I talked to a number of riders who had completed such a ride and decided to sign on for the first "leg" of an XC ride in the summer of 2006, riding from Astoria, OR to Boise, ID. A major learning experience! I came back from that ride with the realization that I could accomplish an XC ride but I would have to change my training, make it more intense (including spinning classes), and change a lot of my equipment.

I left my part-time position in neuroradiology in the spring of 2007 to permit more training miles. With 61 other riders committed to the entire cross-country route, I commenced the fully supported XC ride (America by Bicycle, Plaistow, NH) in mid-June 2007 at Astoria, OR, and 50 days later we were in Portsmouth, NH. Aside from a chronically tender posterior, the "bod" held up well. On such a ride, adequate caloric intake is key. Abundant western-style breakfasts included oatmeal, eggs, potatoes, etc. Rest stops provided bananas, Fig Newtons or other cookies, trail mix and power bars. Lunch on the road might be a Subway stop for a sub sandwich and a soft drink (I didn't worry about soft drinks being "diet"). Dinners were very often at buffet-type restaurants with mega-quantities of salad, pasta, chicken, veggies and desserts. Despite taking in thousands of calories more than usual during the ride, I lost 8 lbs. by the time I arrived in NH. Since completion of the ride, I have managed to gain back most of those pounds lost.

Most people I encounter seem amazed that a 69-year-old male can complete a bike ride across the country. I was the second-oldest in the group, but the oldest to complete the ride (one fellow slightly older than I had to drop out with a knee problem in South Dakota). The combination of maintaining better physical fitness than most men my age through routine exercise (daily), maintaining my weight over the years (weighed 165 lbs. on graduation from college and weighed 169 lbs. at the start of the ride), and solid preparation in terms of training, equipment and nutrition made for the successful completion of the ride. Plus a large dose of good luck, as disaster on a ride such as this is only a pothole away.

Speaking of nutrition, my diet does not include dietary supplements, only a solitary multivitamin. Breakfast is usually orange juice, cold cereal and fruit or oatmeal and a piece of whole wheat toast with homemade preserves (no butter). Lunch is a sandwich or crackers and cheese, yogurt or perhaps soup. Dinners might be pasta, fish (especially here in the NW), an omelet or the very occasional hamburger or steak. My only prescription medicine is an anti-hypertension drug. I became hypertensive about ten years ago, as did my mother. Job stress may have contributed to some degree, but it is probably genetic to large degree.

So, is there a secret to my being able to ride my bike across the country, ski, run and play tennis at an age when many of my colleagues are limited to golf, bridge or television? There is nothing magical at work here. I think the keys are as follows: (1) making physical activity part of my daily routine for as long as I can remember; (2) maintaining my weight with little weight gain over 50 years; (3) eating a healthy diet, and being blessed with a wife with amazing culinary skills who has prepared appetizing, nutritious meals for the past 38 years; (4) good fortune – I have sustained a number of injuries in the course of biking, skating and skiing, but none that could not improve with real medical intervention or tincture of time; and (5) being blessed with good genes.

Thanks, Doc. Not only are you setting an example for other doctors to stay fit, but the general public too. I'm sure they will be glad to see a doctor who practices what he preaches.

HELEN ZACCARIUS

Before I even begin to interview HELEN ZACCARIUS, I have to congratulate this sprightly stepping woman with the beautiful Mediterranean blue eyes who seems way younger than her 69 years on her zest for life as she so actively moves with every step. But she wasn't always this fit. After having three children, she suddenly became very heavy and lost that lively step. She continued to exercise but at five foot five and over 150 pounds, she became grossly out of shape and could not get back to her original size four; although she was still very active, she never ate right.

I never had a weight problem in Greece because I walked everywhere. (And of course hadn't had my children then.) Don't get me wrong: I'm not blaming my weight gain on my children. It's just I didn't think of myself then and as a result, I was eating very badly. I went to many doctors and different places to try and get into shape and lose weight, but nothing seemed to work. I really got very depressed because nothing was Khelping me, so I went to the library and got as many books as I could find on fitness, health and nutrition. (Tony's book wasn't out then.) I guess I was about 48 years of age when I started doing this.

I completely changed my eating habits, and this really seemed to make a difference. I continued to exercise and now that I was eating better, everything seemed to fall into place. I do a lot of swimming and a lot of walking. Almost daily I will work out on the stationary bike. I have eliminated all white foods (sugar, white bread and anything with white flour). I read this in one of the nutrition books. I eat mostly just fish and chicken, and have small portions about five times a day. If I have a sweet dessert I will only take a bite

143

out of it, and that satisfies my yen for it. I do not take any medications but do use vitamins, C-D-E and a calcium supplement. Since I have maintained this program (over twenty years now), I have not had to see a doctor. This almost-69-year-old body feels more like a forty-year-old, and I will continue this regimen because I plan to see my grandchildren grow up.

Great job, Helen. You have proved it's never too late to start a program, and I certainly see the results of the hard work and perseverance you have shown. I see that very lively step that you stated you once had, and you still have the beautiful blue eyes. I know you will see your grandchildren grow up.

CHAPTER SEVEN

YOU ARE WHAT YOU EAT

Let's concentrate on living longer because we want to have a better life. Bombarded with fast food, ethnic food, low carb/high carb, and all the food experts, "YOU ARE WHAT YOU EAT" is a known fact. Food is the fuel that feeds our body to have it run smoothly. Proper foods will assure that you greet the day with the energy to focus, exercise and stay healthy. Even more important is keeping a journal of what you eat each day. As you begin to itemize your intake, you will be amazed at what you actually "shoveled" into your mouth.

Hopefully, as you go along, you will establish the calories of the foods you eat and keep a daily count. The more active you are, the more calories you can take in – but remember it's not just the calories, it's the types of foods that you eat, and what's really important are the portions. You want to pick out the most nutritious foods to keep your energy up. At the end of the book I will list some of the foods that are the most beneficial, according to experts in that field.

Experts say that no more than 30% of your weekly calories should be fat intake. Of course, simply said, you should eliminate as much fat and sugar as possible. Every meal should contain protein, vegetables, fruits, some carbohydrates and whole grains. I personally have eliminated white bread, sugar and anything containing white flour. This can present a problem at times, but should you take the "whites," use very sparingly. If you eat meat, make it very lean and try not to have it too often. I have it about once a week and will have fish and chicken the other days, and of course have moderate portions. I used to eat about three times the amount I now eat; now I eat very small portions but more often. Most experts agree on the fact that we should eat about five times a day. (I was doing this well before I read about it.) This spreads the fuel and you have more energy throughout the day.

Another very important factor in your eating habits: Eat slowly and chew your food thoroughly. Drink plenty of water and try and have something, even if only a fruit, at least every three to four hours. This will keep your metabolism working. Whenever I play ball I always bring nuts, raisins and Fig Newtons with me and eat them during the two games that we play. Originally most of the ball players laughed at this, but now most all of them take some when offered to them.

Gary Null, the noted nutritionist and author of many health books, stated, "You should eat like a king at breakfast, a prince or princess at lunch and a pauper at dinner." I totally agree with him, and why wouldn't I agree with such a notable author.

I recently read the book *Bible Foods*, published by Clarion Call Marketing, 2005. This book stated the Bible foods were the most important foods for our healthy existence. They named garlic, honey, wheat, barley, pomegranate, rice, dates, olives and figs as the Bible foods. I guess God really knew what he was talking about… That sounds pretty good to me, and why wouldn't we listen to God? I know I do. Just a note about figs, which I love and do eat them often: they do contain sugar, but if you eat one you will actually feel the energy that you get from them and they move very quickly through your digestive system. (Get it?) I try to have a couple every day and I will back up that they are a very high source of energy. I'm constantly moving, playing ball three times a week and bowling twice a week, am constantly exercising and am never tired. So I must be doing something right.

When we go dancing, I have to find young girls to go

out with us (my wife's very liberal) because I will tire out all the older women at our table. I'm not bragging; I'm just trying to impress upon you how important it is to eat right and exercise and be active. Dancing is a great aerobic exercise and my favorite.

Another thing is you have to believe in yourself and have a happy attitude. Remember this: It's easier to laugh than frown – frowning causes wrinkles. Do you want wrinkles? I don't.

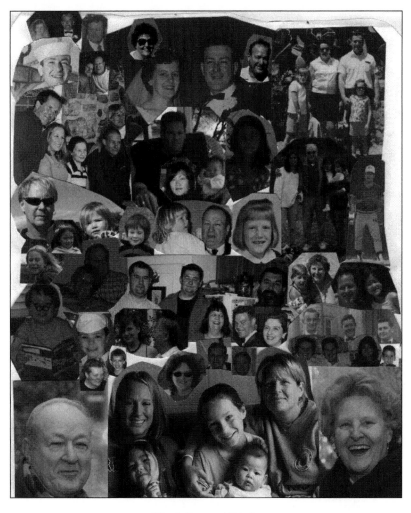

The Author and Family

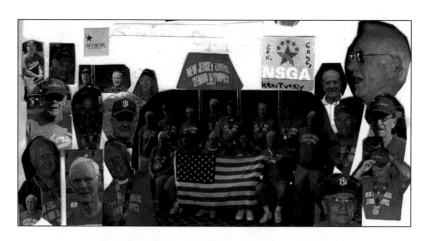

N. J. Senior Olympics team winning the gold medal in the 75-80 division softball team in Louisville, Kentucky, 2007

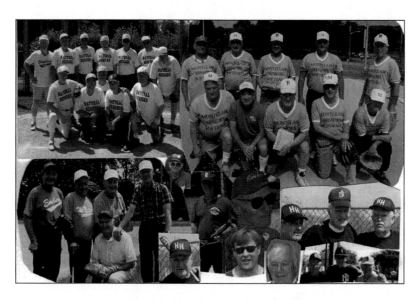

The Naturale's 70 and over senior softball team

CHAPTER EIGHT

MY FIELD OF DREAMS

As author Martin Golan said, "A novel is like a marriage. A short story is like a brief but intense affair. And a poem is like a one night-stand." But I say interviews with people from all walks of life, of all ages, beginning at the ripe old age of seventeen and spanning four score and seven years, is more than a collection of short stories. Hence, MY FIELD OF DREAMS.

As I have reached the ever-young age of 77, time, weather and staying fit have become my best friends, allowing me – if there is no snow on the ground – to greet the day as ever young, still slowing down to a gallop but nonetheless "running" around the bases and playing four to five games a week on the sand lots in my area.

As a senior citizen, I often ask myself, "Self, what would you want to do if you were still a young man?" The answer always comes back to "baseball."

I loved the game so much when I was a kid that I fantasized playing with the New York Giants (now the San Francisco Giants). What does that have to do with fitness? Are you kidding? Not only are you moving your body and enjoying it, but I am out there with other men in my age group who have knee replacements, arthritis, you name it; but we show up because we feel good playing a boy's game. It keeps us young. The field calls to us like a siren and it becomes alive when we show up. Endorphins kick in; we put the cleats on, open the trunks. Suddenly all the aches and pains disappear. We are rubbing shoulders with our youth and we, as a team, will deliver and are an inspiration to each other in a glance, in our silence every time we step up to bat. It's all for one and the camaraderie is unequaled. There are no heroes on this field of dreams. Everyone is just trying to be fit and we meet people from all walks of life.

As one of the ball players stated in his interview, "I wish I could have met you friends years ago." Well, Tom, we're all here now, so let's play ball.

You might have noticed by now that many of the comments about fitness were from my fellow teammates... that was no accident. Many of my fellow seniors are in very good shape. All are playing a kid's game and staying physically fit, just so we can play ball and not injure ourselves.

To everything there is a season but, for now, our "Field of Dreams" – staying fit, thinking like a kid and playing ball – is forever. It doesn't matter who wins the game. If we play the game, we are all winners.

And that means "you."

SUMMARY

"Eat right and exercise." How many times have you heard that? It's not as easy as it sounds. It takes willpower, knowledge of the correct foods, perseverance, and the continuance of all of these.

Well, no one said it would be easy, did they? I'm saying it *will* be easy. You just have to believe in yourself, set goals and just do it. You have to trick your mind and get the right habits. Right now you have eating habits, but are you overweight? If you are, you have to change those habits. It's actually not as hard as you think. You start out slowly with changing just one of the bad habits, and then another and another, and before you know it you will have all the right habits.

I said you have to trick your mind. There are many ways to do that. I will tell you what some of the things were that I did. I'm sitting in the den watching television and I get hungry. I get down and do ten push-ups. What happens? Your hunger disappears – you've tricked your mind. Well, maybe my mind is easier to trick than yours, but I think you get the general idea. And if ten push-ups isn't enough, do more. I have done as many as 100 push-ups (I was very hungry) at times to take away the hunger. It has a dual effect: you're getting in better shape as you get hungrier. You don't always have to do push-ups; try eating an apple or carrot. Eat it slowly and chew it many times. See, you have tricked your mind into not being hungry. You may be a little sore, but you won't be hungry. Many people will drink a glass of water when they get hungry. The secret is if you get hungry and it's not meal time, try eating something of

151

value, like apples, nuts, raisins, etc. YOU HAVE TO GET YOUR MIND OFF OF FOOD.

There are many facets to getting fit. We know you have to eat right and exercise, but you must also get the proper sleep and have a proper state of mind. By that I mean keep the stress down and have a good attitude. Be happy – smile and the world smiles with you.

But most of all, make some attempt to get fit. As I've stated earlier, movement is the key for the fitness equation, so get moving. Be active, have faith and believe in yourself. You will find that everything else will fall into place.

HINT: MOST IMPORTANT – LOG WHAT YOU DO AND WHAT YOU EAT.

I hope many of you reading this book can get something out of the cross-section of people that I have interviewed, as well as some of the things that I do, to help you get ideas for things to do to get active and get in shape. We can all learn from each other. And remember, it's never too late to get started. I know I have learned just from the interviews. So now let's all get started and shape up. See you all on your "Field of Dreams."

EPILOGUE

I would like to end this book by quoting one of our great presidents, ABRAHAM LINCOLN (who was in great shape – and no, I didn't interview him). He very aptly said, "IT'S NOT THE YEARS IN YOUR LIFE THAT COUNT, IT'S THE LIFE IN YOUR YEARS."

And I say:

"THIS IS NOT THE END; THIS IS THE BEGINNING OF A NEW AND HEALTHY YOU." And I don't know who said this but I agree with it: "LIVE WELL, LAUGH OFTEN AND LOVE MUCH, BUT MOST OF ALL BELIEVE IN YOURSELF."

And remember this: "YOU DON'T STOP LAUGHING WHEN YOU GET OLD, YOU GET OLD WHEN YOU STOP LAUGHING…"

Before I end this, I have to tell you this story: I just heard two of the old-time ball players talking. One says to the other, and I quote, "I've sure gotten old! I've had two bypass surgeries, a hip replacement, new knees, fought prostate cancer and diabetes. I'm half blind, can't hear anything quieter than a jet engine, take 40 different medications that make me dizzy, winded, and subject to blackouts. Have bouts with dementia. Have poor circulation; can hardly feel my hands and feet anymore. Can't remember if I'm 85 or 92, and have lost a lot of my friends, but thank God, I'm still playing softball." (Anything sound familiar, guys?)

I would like to thank all of the people that I have interviewed and especially my dear wife, Madeline, who has endured me all these years, living with this fitness nut.

And thank you again, my former agent and long-time friend, author Grange Peggy Habermann, for editing and pushing me to finish this book.

I have found out that I have learned from each and every one of you interviewed with your wonderful inspirational stories. But most of all, thank you, GOD, for allowing me to believe in myself and live the life that I have had. If I had to do it all over again, I would do it exactly as it happened. God bless all of us, and I'll see you all on *my* "Field of Dreams."

THE BEGINNING...

—Anthony Victor Naturale

(Natch)

FOOD LIST

SOME OF THE GOOD FOODS, ACCORDING TO MANY EXPERTS IN THE FIELD, EVEN ME (listed in alphabetical order).

Apples, apricots, asparagus, broccoli, beets, bananas, beans, blackberries, blueberries, cabbage, carrots, cauliflower, celery, chicken, cinnamon, cranberries, egg whites, cold-water fish, figs, garlic, guava, kale, kiwi, lemons, melons, nuts, oats, olives, oranges, peppers, pineapples, prunes, plums, pomegranate juice, pumpkin seeds, pursine (according to researchers at the University of Texas, has the highest amount of heart-healthy omega-3 fats of any edible plant, and I don't even know what that is), raisins, rhubarb, sardines, spinach, strawberries, tomatoes, and don't forget green tea.

There are many others, but these are some of the basic ones and if you stick to the plant foods, you can't go wrong.

Vitamins:

I feel if you eat the proper foods, you don't need too many vitamins. But I am an advocate of certain ones like C, E, B12 and a multivitamin. I also take fish oil, CQ10 and zinc supplements daily. I do use the herb oregano and will use stevia or honey in place of sugar. If I do any heavy lifting of weights, I will take a protein powder, but that's not on a daily basis.

Some of the herbs I will use: oregano, cinnamon, and Echinacea if I feel a cold coming on.

SOME OF THE WORST FOODS:

Butter, bleached white flour, white bread, salt, sugar, sausage, all sodas, french fries, macaroni, cookies, custards, cold cuts, cheese, hot dogs, bacon, butter, creams and any processed and fried foods.

If you eat meat, you should have it very lean and not too often. There are many more bad foods, but these are some of the main ones.

SOURCES

The Internet

The Bible Foods, Clarion Call Marketing, 2005

100 New Natural Cures, Bottom Line Books, 2006.

AARP, the magazine & health section, 2006

Doctor Donald Slocum, PhD, author, lecturer, inventor and ball player

Doctor Michael Kelly, orthopedic surgeon, author

Doctor Alan Williams, MD and cyclist

John Reynolds, physician assistant, holistic expert

Diane Tobin, licensed physical trainer

Gary Null, PhD, author and lecturer (his book: *Natural Healing*, 2004)

Prevention's Best Healing Herbs by the editors of Prevention Health Books, 2001

Barbara Grieco, physical education teacher and author of *The Medical Notebook*

Grange (Peggy) Rutan Habermann, author of *Death of a Bebop Wife* (and my former agent)

Anthony Victor Naturale (me), author of *"YOU'LL NEVER BELIEVE IT"* and *"NATURALE'S LET'S TALK FITNESS CHRONICLES"*, licensed fitness nut (LFN) and retired "half a donut" cop and ballplayer (well, I do have a license)

FOR COMMENTS PLEASE EMAIL Poppopnatch@AOL. com....OR Anthonynatch@optonline.net